Praise for *Whole Body Vibration for Calming Inflammation*

I have been researching whole body vibration (WBV) for years, along with my three brothers, all of whom are also doctors, some of them surgeons. Becky Chambers is the expert; she is very knowledgeable and can guide you on how to use this remarkable system. If you use WBV, go slow and stick with it; then you will see the light at the end of the tunnel. Chronic illness, inflammation, pain, depression, and anxiety can improve because vibration releases stress by changing hormone levels, such as serotonin, cortisol, and endorphins in your brain that are connected to stress, inflammation, pain, and your emotional state. My brothers are amazed at my progress—now they want their own machines!

I am sixty-four years old and have struggled for years with a lot of joint pain. I have now been using Becky's vibration machine and following her advice for the last year. I quickly gained energy and felt stronger, both mentally and physically. Pain and inflammation decreased a lot, and I have been able to stop taking pain killers.

I also have severe osteoporosis. In this last, year my bone density has also improved 29 percent in my hip and femoral neck, according to yearly DEXA scans. In addition, I initially had a large, complex, and potentially carcinogenic cyst on my kidney. This cyst has now shrunk in the last year to only a small simple cyst, which is no longer a cancer risk. Of course, before trying WBV you should check the contraindications and with your doctor and follow their advice.

These machines are indeed a beacon of hope. I feel safer now, because this machine protects me.

—Luz Peguero, MD, age 64

This book, *Whole Body Vibration for Calming Inflammation*, is a jewel of years of research and experience. Combining clinical evidence and guidelines, Becky details the use of whole body vibration (WBV) to calm the harmful effects of inflammation on the body; WBV therapy is taking medical science and technology to a new level.

It's evidence-based fact that inflammation is the driver behind most, if not all, chronic diseases and obesity, creating a channel for effective treatment for clinicians and patients.

Personally, I can attest to the efficacy of WBV in calming inflammation, the major factor in the pain and morbidity that accompany arthritic conditions. I strongly recommend this book as a "must-read" for all, but especially for persons battling chronic disease and/or obesity. It's definitely going on my "read list" for my patients.

It's amazing to find someone like Becky, who has such passion and expertise in this area of medical technology. Congratulations, Becky, on your hard work and effort to help others on the journey to better health and happiness.

—Jean C. Green-Blair, ARNP, clinician
Board Certified Diabetes Care and
Education Specialist (CDCES)
Florida Department of Health, DeSoto County

I am impressed with how thorough yet easy to read this book is, presenting complex information about whole body vibration (WBV) in an accessible and easy-to-read style. I intend to recommend this book and WBV therapy to my associates, and suggest to my clients that they read it. I feel sure that then they will have all the information they need, not only about WBV but all of the supporting lifestyle [changes] necessary for the best results as well. I am also impressed by how many issues a WBV practice addresses!

Becky is right, WBV has powerful effects all throughout your body, including [reducing] inflammation and detoxification—I was overenthusiastic the first day that I used the platform. I did seven minutes, thinking, "Oh, this is no big deal." Boy was I wrong! Twenty-four hours later every muscle in my body hurt! I remembered Becky's book and took charcoal and began to have relief within twenty minutes. I am grateful for the information in this book; it is deeply helpful, especially for stubborn know-it-all's!

—Rain Juvoli, ND, retired

Becky Chambers's new book, *Whole Body Vibration for Calming Inflammation*, is a must read for almost any health-care provider, as well as anyone suffering from pain or chronic inflammation. Whole body vibration (WBV) has a place in osteoarthritis, gut health, and chronic pain, amongst many other health challenges. In this book, she has compiled the latest research on WBV, showing weight loss, increased bone density, and muscle strength, along with decreasing pain and inflammation.

Research has shown that low back pain, fibromyalgia, and knee osteoarthritis can all be addressed with WBV.

What is even better is that the book has easy-to-implement protocols that almost anyone can incorporate into their day-to-day routine or into their health-care practice. From pain reduction to exercise, and anti-inflammatory protocols to purchasing the right type of vibration plate, this new book has it all. This is the best book I have ever read on whole body vibration.

—Dr. Lee E. Zohn, DAAPM, CCSP
Chiropractic physician

I have been able to see firsthand the benefits of whole body vibration for my clients as well as myself. After careful research to find the best vibration platform that would deliver the most effective and gentle vibration for my clients and patients, I found the Power 1000 via Becky Chambers and her company Vibrant Health. My clients love it! I have patients that are improving their bone density after treatment for breast cancer. Many others are recovering their balance and strength after cancer treatment. And others are reducing inflammation and painful swelling in their bodies. Even clients who have had swelling in the legs for over twenty years from old injuries have had dramatic reductions in swelling that is sustainable using WBV. I can say WBV helped me lose "that last ten pounds." It totally lifts my mood as well.

Becky has done a wonderful job of disseminating the research to provide clear instruction on how to effectively use WBV. She has taken a deep dive into why and how it works so you can be confident in your treatment plan. She has provided a wonderful guide in this book for you to begin to change your life with WBV. Chronic inflammation is at the root of most disease processes of our modern lifestyle. Tools like WBV that can reduce inflammation have tremendous potential to impact our quality of life and health.

—Lisa Moore PT, DPT, CLT
Owner of Reach Cancer Rehab and Wellness
www.ReachCancerRehabandWellness.com
Tacoma, WA

Becky Chambers has clearly emerged as one of the most experienced experts on whole body vibration (WBV). Becky has written a scientifically based book that is inspiring and easy to read.

Not only will you become excited to add WBV to your life, but you will also have a far deeper understanding of how it works and why it works. People truly get remarkable results.

I love my WBV practices, and I recommend them to my patients as well. Easily, it is one of the most effective and efficient ways to exercise, deflame, and detoxify.

—Jonathan Glass, MAc, Ayurvedic practitioner
author of *The Total Life Cleanse*

Becky Chambers's new book, *Whole Body Vibration for Calming Inflammation*, presents exciting research findings to reduce inflammation, improve the intestinal microbiome, and combat chronic disease such as metabolic syndrome and type 2 diabetes with the use of whole body vibration (WBV). Her own research and the findings of other respected studies establishes the benefit of WBV for improving osteoporosis, inflammation, and pain. Even greater improvements are realized when combined with other proven therapies. Becky Chambers is truly leading the way for people who want to enjoy a healthy life!

My ninety-six-year-old mother, who has heart failure and COPD, quickly becomes tired and short of breath when walking or exercising. However, she definitely enjoys using her Vibrant Health Gentle 500 vibration machine twice each day to stay in shape. She happily reports more energy and less pain in her knees (without any shortness of breath) after using her WBV machine, and she can keep on gardening, which she loves!

I have found that frequent use of my larger Vibrant Health WBV machine relieves the chronic pain in my sacrum and coccyx, remnants of a disabling injury [sustained] while serving in the US Navy.

—Teresa McFarland, RN, MSN, FNP-C
Commander, Navy Nurse Corps, USN (retired)

Becky Chambers has already proven herself as one of the leading experts in the field of whole body vibration. The most recent research she writes about in her new book addressing inflammation and improvements in gut health using whole body vibration is innovative and cutting edge. I am looking forward to implementing whole body vibration into my practice in the future.

—Dr. Blanki Cherunini MD, FAAPMR
Intervention & Functional Pain Center

If you are curious about whole body vibration (WBV), Becky Chambers is the master of this healing tool. In this book, she has gathered the most recent research on the health benefits of WBV for optimizing our immune system, reducing inflammation, and other timely concerns that challenge us. This concise, easy-to-read book will show you how to use this therapeutic exercise system for optimal health and healing, encouraging our bodies to age gracefully.

—Barry Taylor, ND
author of *Love Your Body: Your Path
to Transformation, Health and Healing* and
creator of Love Your Body online workshops
www.DrBarry@DrBarryTaylor.com

Whole body vibration has been a great support, both for myself and for many of my clients. Becky's machines are the best. . . . I tried several before I found hers. Becky's passion to share her research, knowledge, and excitement about this modality is reflected once again in this latest book on WBV's ability to quell inflammation.

—Bonnie Grace
Registered physical therapist
Certified Feldenkrais practitioner

Becky clearly explains how whole body vibration (WBV) can begin a cascade of positive responses within the body to keep inflammation low and improve long-term health. Teaching our patients how to manage inflammation can greatly impact their quality of life.

I co-own a wellness center with a chiropractor, Dr. Jeanette Wilburn, in Western Massachusetts, where we use WBV as an adjunct to multiple services. Reading this book has not only reinvigorated me to expand our in-clinic utilization of WBV but also to get on mine at home every day. Thank you, Becky.

—Stephanie Nascimento, RN, CA

Also by Becky Chambers

*Whole Body Vibration for Mental Health:
Natural Methods for Finding Peace Amid Chaos*

Whole Body Vibration for Seniors

*Homeopathy Plus Whole Body Vibration:
Combining Two Energy Medicines Ignites Healing*

*Whole Body Vibration:
The Future of Good Health*

Whole Body Vibration
for Calming Inflammation

Becky Chambers, BS, MEd

The Global Authority on Vibration Therapy
and author of the best-selling book
Whole Body Vibration: The Future of Good Health

Transformations

Copyright © 2022 by Becky Chambers, BS, MEd

All rights reserved, including the right to reproduce this work in any form whatsoever, without permission in writing from the author, except for brief passages in connection with a review.

This book is written as a source of information to educate the readers. It is not intended to replace medical advice or care, whether provided by a primary care physician, specialist, or other health-care professional, including a licensed alternative medical practitioner. Please consult your doctor if you are experiencing any symptoms that scare or concern you and before beginning any form of health program. Neither the author nor the publisher shall be liable or responsible for any adverse effects arising from the use or application of any of the information contained herein, nor do they guarantee that everyone will benefit or be healed by these techniques or practices, nor are they responsible if individuals do not so benefit.

Cover design by Darryl Khalil
Interior design by Jane Hagaman
Model in exercise section: Ula Zielinska
Model photos by Rick Dorrington
Author photo by Miranda Loud

Published by Transformations
Lexington, MA

If you are unable to order this book from your local bookseller, you may order directly from the author at her website: BCVibrantHealth.com.

Library of Congress Control Number: 2021920019

ISBN 978-0-9890662-8-0
10 9 8 7 6 5 4 3 2 1

Printed on acid-free paper in the United States

To my much appreciated clients and customers,
whose success and enthusiasm give me strength
and make my work worth the effort.

Contents

Foreword, by Dr. Peter Bongiorno — xvii
Preface — xxi
Acknowledgments — xxv
Introduction. What If? — xxvii

CHAPTER 1
Your Natural Anti-Inflammation Plan — 1

CHAPTER 2
Introduction to Whole Body Vibration — 11

CHAPTER 3
Cutting-Edge Inflammation Research — 25

CHAPTER 4
Whole Body Vibration and Pain — 39

CHAPTER 5
Losing Weight with Whole Body Vibration — 49

CHAPTER 6
A Healthy Gut = A Calm Immune System — 65

CHAPTER 7
A Quick and Easy Anti-Inflammation Food Plan — 77

Chapter 8
Balancing Gut Flora   93

Chapter 9
Detoxing with Whole Body Vibration   113

Chapter 10
Exercise   125

Chapter 11
Meditation, Yoga, and Other Therapies to Reduce Stress   131

Chapter 12
Choosing a Whole Body Vibration Machine   137

Chapter 13
Getting Started with Whole Body Vibration   161

Appendix 1. Vibrant Health Research Survey Summary   177

Appendix 2. Brain Synchronization   187

Appendix 3. FODMAP Diet Foods   191

Appendix 4. Severe *Candida* Yeast Overgrowth   193

Appendix 5. Contraindications   197

Notes   201

Resources, Suggested Reading, and Additional Research
   Studies   215

Foreword

The impressionist artist Monet painted haystacks, and more haystacks. He painted them over and over—in diverse lighting, in various weather cover, and at different times of day. He artfully brought the viewer a matchless understanding of not only haystacks themselves but also of color, light, the brilliance of nature itself. The observing art lover also found a profound change in their own perspective of the world.

Becky Chambers is another such artist, and vibrational medicine is her haystack. The book you are holding represents her fifth book on the subject. And each of her books takes a different perspective regarding this growing movement in health. A movement she fearlessly leads. In each successive book, she delves deeper and more significantly into the fundamentals of health itself as it relates to whole body vibration. As a result, we, as the readers, can view our health in a different way and learn to heal ourselves in the process.

Having been in practice for nearly two decades in New York and having authored seminal books on the subject of mental health, I have deeply investigated the underlying causes of mental health disorders, and I have learned that we need all hands on deck when dealing with illness. What works for one person may not work for another. And sometimes healing comes in a form that is not always expected—or intuitive.

In my patients' quest for healing over time, many have brought to me for my opinion the latest health "breakthroughs." I have seen many of these come and go. I have fielded questions for this perfect new diet, that latest miracle vitamin, and the newest detox cure. If you have not heard of vibrational therapy, at first glance you may think it's another one of those breakthroughs that, upon first glance, might come and go, too.

In this book, Becky Chambers teaches us that, like Monet's haystacks, looking at this modality of treatment from yet another viewpoint and light only reinforces the solid research and physiology that she has taught us in her past books on the subject. She demonstrates to us once again that vibrational therapy is not going away anytime soon and is gaining ground in both the scientific literature and the clinical community.

In *Whole Body Vibration for Calming Inflammation*, Ms. Chambers takes on a pathological behemoth: inflammation. Conventional care views eczema, joint pain, autoimmune disease, digestive dysfunction, obesity, cardiovascular disease, and even cancer as disparate problems to be treated with immune suppressive medications, acid blockers, appetite suppressants, statin drugs, and chemotherapy respectively. What modern medicine hasn't quite figured out is that inflammation is the fundamental underlying cause of most illness.

Ms. Chambers's latest work takes on the inflammatory cascade by teaching us that this not-so-novel modality can indeed balance inflammation. It does this by a few mechanisms: it can calm the stress system, improve gut function, and even help balance the good bacteria in the digestive tract. These are three potent ways to switch our body system from "flame on" to "flame off." It also gives us clear evidence that upon resolving the inflammation, vibrational therapy will also help initiate regenerative repair. What drug can possibly do that—and with no side effects?

Whole Body Vibration for Calming Inflammation is not a monochromatic painting but, indeed, a three-dimensional representation employing a full-color pallet. Beyond whole body vibration, Ms. Chambers underscores the necessity of nutrition, lifestyle, detoxification, and social connection to remind us that true holistic healing requires a comprehensive plan to help the body heal itself. There are clear and helpful recommendations that are easy to bring into your day. She also tackles some special topics, such as brain synchronization and yeast clearing, to optimize your whole body vibration outcomes.

Take your valuable time and read this book. Keep a pen on hand and jot down what is important to you—there is so much good information, you will want to keep track of what you find most beneficial for your care.

Ms. Chambers proposes that "WBV makes you feel alive—ten minutes, and your body will be tingling head to toe." Take this as your challenge and find out for yourself how it can make you feel. Find out why Becky Chambers's books are gaining more ground and attention with each iteration. Realize at a deeper level how the body can heal itself. And most of all, see how this latest "haystack" in Becky Chambers's library can give you a new powerful perspective on your health by lowering inflammation.

—Dr. Peter Bongiorno
naturopathic doctor and acupuncturist;
past president, New York Association
of Naturopathic Physicians, www.nyanp.org
www.drpeterbongiorno.com
(also on Facebook, Instagram, and Twitter)

Author of:
*Holistic Solutions for Anxiety and Depression:
Combining Natural Remedies with Conventional Care*

*How Come They're Happy and I'm Not?
The Complete Natural Program for Healing Depression for Good*

*Put Anxiety Behind You:
The Complete Drug-Free Program*
(Natural Relief from Anxiety, for Readers of Dare)

Preface

I am a classic "canary in the mine." At the age of fifteen, my body began rebelling against the stresses of modern life by developing a host of health issues linked to chronic inflammation. Those issues started when I was a young child with depression, which became severe at times, and continued for thirty years. I developed addictive and emotional eating behaviors, including bulimia, and ate all the wrong foods. By my early twenties, I weighed two hundred pounds. By then, I also had rampant food sensitivities, painful digestive symptoms, immune system weakness, and numerous disabling joint and nervous system problems—classic signs of inflammation. Back then, I was an isolated freak of nature; today, my experiences are becoming commonplace as chronic inflammation and chronic health issues skyrocket.

The field of chronic illness is vast and still uncharted. Many people find that they need to go beyond standard allopathic (conventional) medicine to holistic healers, acupuncturists, homeopaths, chiropractors, herbalists, functional medicine practitioners, integrative medicine physicians, and naturopathic physicians to find a path through the forest—or rather the jungle—back to good health.

Having developed chronic illnesses at a young age, I have four decades of experience with healing myself. I threw a wide net when seeking help. I received guidance from practitioners and researchers in all of the above fields.

Then twenty years ago, along came whole body vibration, which for me turned out to be the linchpin for stimulating and strengthening my body and mind, decreasing inflammation and pain, clearing out toxins, and speeding my recovery to where I am today—a vibrant, healthy sixty-two-year-old.

In this book, I share with you my knowledge, my experiences, my research; what has worked and not worked for me and hundreds of my clients over the years. Because I have lived through more than forty years of these issues and found a way to not only survive but also thrive, there is information in this book that you will not find anywhere else.

We all need to appreciate that the field of chronic illness and inflammation is still in the pioneer phase. Information is changing quickly. What I believe and have stressed in these pages is that along with whole body vibration (WBV) technology, we need to return to a more natural and whole way of eating and living. We need to live mindfully, to be aware of what we are eating, to slow down, and to have gratitude and appreciation for our natural world, the life we live, and the people in our lives. We need to love more and appreciate the interconnectivity of all beings.

And we need to be open to the many alternatives to allopathic medicine, which has its place and can be important and useful, but buyer beware if you are relying only on allopathic medicine and drugs to heal your chronic illness. Do not blindly follow a system of medicine that has been compromised by drug profiteering.

I give a lot of credit to Dr. DeOrio, my now-retired medical doctor, who was an early proponent of WBV, a homeopath, and a natural health medical doctor, and to the many other health-care professionals who have contributed to my knowledge and success. But I am the one who has lived through this, and there is no teacher like personal experience. I have spent at least 100,000 hours researching and trying different methods in the pursuit of a path to healing. Now, with the millions of people suffering issues similar to those that I have been dealing with all my life, it feels as if I am meant to share my knowledge.

When I first found WBV and felt nearly instant relief, I was excited and planned to incorporate this technology into my own natural health-care practice. This plan had a slow start, as machines at that time cost $10,000 or more and nobody had heard of WBV. In the end, that slow start was good, as those big, expensive machines are not the right ones for people with health issues. Five years after first trying WBV, I had learned much, had the proper type of machine, and the cost had come down. The time was right to reach out to a larger audience, so I began to use WBV with other people and to write about WBV. This is my fifth book on the subject.

Acknowledgments

I want to especially thank my clients, for teaching me and encouraging me with their successes and struggles. The work cannot be done without you! Special thanks to those who provided personal testimonials for this book.

Many health-care professionals have contributed to my journey to health and knowledge, and I thank them all for their hard work and help along my path. Particular thanks go to Keith DeOrio, MD (retired), who was a leader in recognizing the potential of whole body vibration in health care and taught me much about this technology and other natural health approaches.

Writing a book is a challenging process; many thanks to all those who help me with their excellent professional help. Thank you, Jeanne Mayell, content editor; Tania Seymour, copy editor; Jane Hagaman, interior book designer; and Darryl Khalil, cover designer. I would also like to thank Dr. Jack Yu for his support and encouragement and careful technical review of this book.

Thank you also to my family and friends, who give me love and joy—a beautiful and cherished gift.

Introduction

What If?

What if there were a natural and safe way to lower inflammation? What if when you were given a diagnosis of diabetes, or high blood pressure, or IBS (irritable bowel syndrome), or any of the numerous other inflammation-driven chronic health conditions, your doctor told you that *you could heal yourself*, that you do not need to take potentially dangerous drugs for the rest of your life. That day is coming, and whole body vibration, with its booming popularity and long list of health benefits, including lowering inflammation, is leading the way.

In today's world, where stress and other lifestyle factors have led to high rates of chronic diseases linked to inflammation and the transmission of infectious viruses and other diseases can be breathtakingly rapid and potentially deadly, keeping your health and immune system in top working order is a must. Rather than depending on drugs that just put a bandage on the problem while causing more problems elsewhere and starting a downward slide, the best approach to your health is to calm inflammation and strengthen your body and immune system with natural health methods.

This is where whole body vibration can be a beacon in the darkness. New research is confirming that whole body vibration (WBV) lowers inflammation and invigorates and stimulates your immune system at the same time. How does it do this? By helping your body to do what it does better than any man-made drug will ever be able to do—maintain, heal, and repair itself. WBV gives you the stimulation, on multiple levels (physical, mental, and energetic), that your body was designed to thrive on.

Ten minutes on the vibration plate will feel like you have run a mile. Your blood zings through every blood vessel, your brain lights up, hormones increase, energy and mood rise—all of which boosts your immune system along with other critical aspects of health. WBV makes you feel alive—ten minutes, and your body will be tingling head to toe. It is common sense, especially for people who are sedentary and getting little stimulation, that WBV would be good for your health.

What if, when you went to the doctor, he or she told you to get a vibration machine and learn how to calm the inflammation in your body that is aggravating or causing your health issue? What if you are just beginning the best years of your life? WBV has the potential to help us all turn our lives around.

NOTE: The information in this book is not intended to be a substitute for professional medical advice, diagnosis, or treatment. Always seek the advice of your doctor or other qualified health provider if you have a medical condition or have any questions regarding a medical condition and/or medical symptoms.

Please check the list of whole body vibration contraindications in appendix 5 and consult with your doctor before beginning whole body vibration.

Chapter 1

Your Natural Anti-Inflammation Plan

Almost all chronic health diseases have one thing in common—inflammation. In fact, chronic inflammation is recognized as a driving force in health conditions as diverse as obesity, diabetes, heart disease, hypertension, arthritis, autoimmune diseases, allergies, asthma, Alzheimer's, numerous digestive issues, and others.[1] With more than 50 percent of the adult population suffering with a chronic health condition, according to a 2018 CDC study,[2] if you don't have one yourself, you probably know someone who does. A quick, easy, and safe anti-inflammation method would be revolutionary.

Whole body vibration, an exercise and therapeutic system booming worldwide and used by clinics around the world in the treatment of many conditions, has now also been shown in numerous research studies to decrease inflammation (see chapter 3). This simple, at-home system has the potential to revolutionize health care for millions of people.

Whole body vibration reduces inflammation, plus it has numerous other benefits that will help you follow a healthy lifestyle, which will also help reduce inflammation. For these reasons, whole body vibration (WBV) should be the cornerstone of your anti-inflammation plan. Rapidly and easily,[i] whole body vibration can alleviate inflammation and pain, plus give you energy and a better mood—all of which can help you to build your own powerful, natural, anti-inflammation plan using the methods in this book.

> **Whole body vibration reduces inflammation, plus it has numerous other benefits that will help you follow a healthy lifestyle, which will also help reduce inflammation.**

Using WBV for lowering inflammation is easy. Especially at the beginning, to reduce inflammation and enjoy those other beneficial side effects, all you need to do is stand on your machine for a few minutes each day. I know this seems so simple and easy that it must be too good to be true. But recent research is confirming what I have been seeing and talking about for years.

WBV should be the foundation of your plan, but do not neglect other natural approaches if you seek the best chance of success. A combined approach of WBV plus other natural-health methods will most effectively

---

[i] WBV is powerful, so to avoid overdosing, be sure to follow instructions to start slow, using the lowest speed for only 30–60 seconds; then gradually increase speed and length of time to the extent that your body can easily tolerate—meaning with no aggravation of your symptoms. See chapter 13 for more guidelines on getting started.

eliminate sources of inflammation and bring soothing relief to inflamed tissues.

In the following chapters, I will explain how to best use WBV for reducing inflammation, and I will also give you other natural inflammation-lowering methods. Read through these methods to see which ones appeal to you. Then choose at least six or seven of these methods; one of them must be WBV, and try to also do something for gut health. If you are having trouble getting started, begin with just a little bit of vibration. As you begin to feel better, start adding other methods; then watch what happens as your team of inflammation firefighters work together to put out the flames!

What Is Inflammation?

Inflammation is an essential process of the immune system—it is the result of the immune system attacking "invaders." Acute, short-term, localized inflammation is a healthy, protective process that brings infection-fighting cells and chemicals to areas where they are needed, such as when the body responds to a bug bite, an invading virus or bacteria, or injury. Without this immune system–inflammation response, our bodies would soon be overrun by viruses, bacteria, other toxins, and disease organisms.

> *A combined approach of WBV plus other natural-health methods will most effectively eliminate sources of inflammation and bring soothing relief to inflamed tissues.*

But inflammation can also become a chronic low-grade systemic state that causes damage to tissues throughout the body. For example, blood vessels, such as coronary arteries, and brain tissue can become inflamed, as happens in heart disease and brain diseases. In other situations, such as when the immune system is overwhelmed, stressed, and out of balance, it can get confused and begin attacking benign substances (causing allergies) or your own tissues (causing autoimmune diseases).

Inflammation reactions increase the blood flow to the area of injury or infection, which often causes redness and warmth in these areas. Some of the chemicals released cause fluid to leak into your tissues, resulting in swelling. If there are nerves in the area, such as in joints, this process will cause pain. If there are not any nerves in the area of inflammation, such as is often the case with inflammation of internal organs like the heart, lungs, or kidneys, then you will not feel pain, but there is still damage happening to the tissues.

There is a continuum of chronic inflammation-related health problems from relatively small issues, such as minor digestive symptoms, acne, and allergies; to more serious situations in which the inflammation is causing damage in critical organs like the heart; and finally to autoimmune diseases in which the immune system is so out of whack that it has begun to attack your own body.

PLEASE READ THIS IMPORTANT WARNING: You should always consult with and work with your doctor while trying the methods in this book, especially if you have progressed further along the continuum of inflammation-induced health issues. WBV is not safe or appropriate for severe, acute inflammation, including acute episodes of chronic inflammatory conditions. In these situations, you need to see a doctor and support and calm your body using other methods, including recommended prescription medications, before trying WBV. Please also check the contraindications for WBV on page 197 before beginning WBV.

Causes of Inflammation

Common triggers for chronic inflammation are an unhealthy gut, poor nutrition, trauma and stress, obesity, toxins, and addictions. Your digestive system is where essential nutrients enter the body and where dangerous bacteria, undigested food, and other foreign invaders must be kept out. When this system is not working properly, toxic waste products, foreign particles, undigested food, and other immune-system triggers can leak into your bloodstream, resulting in your immune system going into overdrive trying to defend you, leading to chronic inflammation.

Gut health is critical to reducing inflammation. WBV has several effects that directly improve gut health, from improving gut flora balance and reducing inflammatory cytokines (chemicals produced by the immune system) in the gut to improving your mental attitude so it is easier to control what you eat. Certain diets and foods, nutritional supplements, and lifestyle changes will also help heal and support gut and immune-system health.

Recently, there has been a greater understanding of the role of stress and trauma in chronic inflammation. Physical, mental, or

> *Gut health is critical to reducing inflammation. WBV has several effects that directly improve gut health, from improving gut flora balance and reducing inflammatory cytokines in the gut to improving your mental attitude so it is easier to control what you eat.*

emotional stress will cause an acute stress response in the body, which negatively affects the immune system when it becomes chronic. We have all experienced the adrenalin-rush reaction of a pounding heart, sweaty hands, and heightened awareness that comes with perceived danger. This automatic activation system can be a powerful protective reaction that revs up the body, including the immune system, for action in response to a threat. But when stress is chronic, as it often is in modern life, then the body is chronically in this "fight-or-flight" mode. In this state, the immune system is constantly in attack mode, creating chronic inflammation that leads to an exhausted immune system prone to making errors and a body that is not focused on day-to-day functions such as digestion, healing, and repair.

This same mind-body connection means that the relaxing and de-stressing effects of WBV result in a calming effect on your immune system. WBV feels like a relaxing massage. It increases serotonin and other feel-good neurotransmitters in the brain.[3] This helps to slow and calm your thoughts so your brain can move out of "fight or flight" and into a more meditative state where the body naturally focuses on healing. These effects can be further heightened using methods such as meditation, yoga, and exercise.

Another area in which WBV can help in the battle against inflammation is through weight loss. Obesity has a complex feedback relationship to inflammation where obesity leads to chronic inflammation, and chronic inflammation makes it harder to lose weight. Breaking out of this vicious cycle can be difficult, but WBV can help here as well; WBV has been shown in hundreds of studies to expedite weight loss,[4] especially when combined with diet and other exercise.

> *This same mind-body connection means that the relaxing and de-stressing effects of WBV result in a calming effect on your immune system.*

Toxins are impossible to avoid in the modern world. Thousands of potentially harmful chemicals are in products we use every day in the US, from food to electronics to medical equipment and carpets. Toxins, especially heavy metals, will damage our sensitive immune and nervous systems, disrupting normal functioning. Detoxification is an area in which WBV excels. Just standing on a vibration plate causes all our muscle fibers to tense and relax, which pumps our lymphatic system, thereby moving toxins and other waste products out of our bodies.

Addictions may also be linked to inflammation in a self-perpetuating cycle. Alcohol, certain foods, obesity itself, and

WBV has been shown in hundreds of studies to expedite weight loss, especially when combined with diet and other exercise.

depression can all cause inflammation, but inflammation can also cause depression and increase addictive cravings of all sorts.[5] WBV can help intervene in this cycle by raising serotonin and calming the mind (which can alleviate depression) and by lowering inflammation—and both of these effects can aid in controlling cravings.

There are numerous causes of chronic inflammation, and WBV can assist with many of them, but combining WBV with other natural methods will boost your results.

Read on to find out what else you can do.

Drugs

If you have a chronic health condition, you are likely already taking prescription medication. More than half of Americans now regularly take prescription medication—four different drugs, on average—according to a 2017 *Consumer Reports* survey of 1,947 adults.[6] These drugs are important. They can lower your risk of dangerous outcomes, and they are appealing for their often quick symptomatic relief. But drugs also have side-effects, ranging from irritating to life threatening. Plus, because drugs generally have some level of toxicity and they do not address the root causes of inflammation and poor health, this approach, especially over time, can lead to a disastrous downhill slide of more health issues and more drugs.

What can you do? Fight back with your own natural anti-inflammation plan.

If you are currently on anti-inflammation or other medications, do not stop taking them on your own—this is not a safe thing to try. Consult with your doctor. Let them know you are trying natural methods to help lower your inflammation levels and, if you wish, work with them to try to reduce your medication.

You can also work with a physician who specializes in incorporating natural methods in treatment plans, such as a naturopathic doctor (ND). (Other terms for doctors and approaches that combine natural and Western medicine include functional, integrative, and complementary medicine.) These doctors, or a conventional doctor, can evaluate you for specific risk factors and causes of your symptoms and inflammation (such as levels of inflammatory markers, hormone and nutrient levels, food sensitivities, and gut health). See page 215 for further resources and to find a naturopathic physician or other natural health professional near you.

The beauty of natural health methods is that while safely lowering inflammation, they also have other benefits for your life and health. Natural methods improve the quality of your life. They are also cost effective, saving you money in the long run, as they help you avoid costly medical treatments. And there are rarely negative side effects to natural health methods, only additional positive effects. Many of the methods in this book cost little to nothing. A natural-health approach is a win-win situation with virtually no negatives, only positives, so let's get started.

Chapter 2

Introduction to Whole Body Vibration

The field of whole body vibration is changing; new research is pouring in from all over the world. For the latest research results and developments in the field of whole body vibration, please check my website.

(BCVibrantHealth.com)

Whole body vibration (WBV) should be the foundation of your natural anti-inflammation plan. Whole body vibration works in multiple ways to lower inflammation, from changing levels of key inflammatory immune system cells and cytokines (immune system chemicals) to increasing beneficial gut flora and decreasing stress levels.

Whole body vibration works in multiple ways to lower inflammation, from changing levels of key inflammatory immune system cells and cytokines to increasing beneficial gut flora and decreasing stress levels.

WBV is the lynchpin that can enhance and amplify the other methods suggested in this book. However, like any powerful treatment, it is important to use it correctly: check the contraindications (appendix 5); make sure you are using the right type of machine; and be sure to stop, rest, and reevaluate if any symptoms are worsening—it is possible to overdose on WBV, which can aggravate symptoms (more about these important aspects of vibration later—see chapters 4, 8, 9, 12, and 13). Remember that WBV's effects are global to the whole body. If you have chronic health conditions, be careful not to use too much WBV too quickly.

All vibration machines are not equal: Be sure to do your WBV every day, but do not use just any type of vibration. All vibration is not the same. As I will describe later, to get the best anti-inflammation effect, the vibration machine you use should be synchronized, smooth, and calming; not too strong or chaotic, or the anti-inflammatory effect and some other benefits may not be realized. Vibration is a workout, which is a foundation of health, but synchronized, smooth, calm vibrations can also help your brain to get in sync with an orderly rhythm rather than creating a conflict in your system. Brain synchronization (see also appendix 2) is associated with reduced stress and improved mental health,[ii] another goal of your anti-inflammatory program.

When you stand on a vibration plate, you can feel the vibrations going through your body with a sensation similar to a mas-

---

[ii]There have been many studies to back these claims. Please see the "Brain Synchronization" section under Additional Research Studies at the back of the book.

sage. WBV seems so simple, but every cell and molecule in your body vibrates, leading to a cascade of effects, including calming and balancing your immune and nervous systems. The results of WBV are so global, affecting you from head to toe, that it can be hard to believe. It is true, though, and has been documented during fifty years of research.[1]

Used properly, WBV can bring rapid increases in strength, mobility, and energy, and decreases in pain, as well as other benefits.[2] As pain is closely linked to inflammation, it is not surprising that recent WBV research is now also documenting decreasing inflammation.

My own recent research survey[3] of fifty-three of my customers (out of 187 surveys sent out) also reported large gains in these areas (see appendix 1 for a summary of the survey methods and results). This is particularly significant because 90 percent of my customers and clients are over the age of fifty, and older people with health issues are a population in which good results with WBV are not easily found, as you will see in later discussions of the research on WBV. Clinical trials using my methods should be done to confirm these self-reported survey results, but as a preliminary study, the results are encouraging.

> **WBV seems so simple, but every cell and molecule in your body vibrates, leading to a cascade of effects, including calming and balancing your immune and nervous systems.**

Benefits from Whole Body Vibration

Exercise: WBV is best known as an intense workout system, and exercise itself is well known to bring about anti-inflammatory benefits. In the beginning, or if you are not feeling well, you can simply stand on the gently vibrating plate, receiving a vibration that will feel like a massage. Through the involuntary automatic activation of your nervous system, and thus your muscles, you will still be experiencing a mild workout. At the other end of the spectrum, ten minutes of WBV while holding exercise positions on the plate equals one hour of conventional weightlifting.

At first that idea may seem impossible, just too good to be true, but it is true. While the exact ratio does depend on which machine you use and how you use it (whether you utilize exercise positions or just stand on the plate), fifty years of research and the devotion of thousands of professional athletes and elite users—including Shaquille O'Neil, Jane Fonda, many Olym-

> *In the beginning, you can simply stand on the gently vibrating plate, and through the involuntary automatic activation of your nervous system, you will experience a mild workout. However, ten minutes of WBV while holding exercise positions on the plate equals one hour of conventional weightlifting.*

pic athletes, and other professional sports franchises, such as the Denver Broncos and the Tennessee Titans—can attest to WBV's effectiveness.

Holding different positions while on a vibrating plate will require different muscle groups to hold your body weight against the vibration. For example, when you are in a squat position, your leg muscles have to hold your body weight against the vibration—and this is hard work, much harder than holding this position on the floor. See below for an explanation of why this is so. **Also see chapter 13 for photos of exercise positions you can use while on the vibration plate to target different muscle groups and for guidelines for using WBV for exercise.**

How Whole Body Vibration Creates Intensive Exercise

- ♦ Holding weight against vibration increases the effects of gravity. Because of this physical reality (described mathematically as gravity equals mass times acceleration), when vibrating, your muscles must hold two to three times your actual weight, the exact amount depending on the amplitude of the vibration. If you are in any doubt about this, consider the arm and shoulder muscle development of men who operate jackhammers.

- ♦ Every muscle fiber will automatically tense and relax at the same rate that the machine is vibrating, usually twenty to fifty times per second. That adds up to one thousand to three thousand little tiny "reps" per minute—much more work for your muscles than holding a position (static or isometric exercise) or typical repetition workouts.

- One hundred percent of your muscles will be working, while in traditional exercises, only some of your muscles are engaged. For example, in a nonvibrating squat, only about 40 percent of your leg muscles are working, but if you are vibrating, 100 percent of your leg muscles will be firing.

The workout itself helps promote health and lower inflammation in numerous ways. Increased circulation brings more nutrients and oxygen to cells and removes waste products, which improve cellular healing and functions. Exercise helps you lose weight and calm the mind, both of which have anti-inflammatory effects. Exercise, and WBV (see below), boosts energy, strength, and mental attitude—all of which will help you add more methods and stick to the more difficult ones in this book, such as changing your diet and increasing other exercise as well.

Mental Health and Energy Levels: Two neurotransmitters, serotonin and norepinephrine, have been shown to increase with WBV.[4] Serotonin is an important neurotransmitter in your brain that contributes to sounder sleep and feelings of mastery, pleasure, and relaxation. This is the same neurotransmitter that is targeted by prescription antidepressant drugs such as Prozac and Wellbutrin, as well as marijuana and many Schedule I and II drugs such as heroin, cocaine, and Ecstasy. While prescription drugs for depression can be valuable for helping to alleviate symptoms, they also have side effects, and they can lead to increasing tolerance and dependence on those drugs. Whole body vibration is a natural, safe, rapid, nonaddictive, and legal way to increase serotonin and norepinephrine.

Norepinephrine is both a neurotransmitter and a hormone, and low levels of this essential molecule have been linked to depression and low energy. Norepinephrine (along with epinephrine) underlies the fight-or-flight response, giving the body sudden energy in times of stress; it increases the heart rate, triggers the release of glucose from energy stores, increases blood flow to skeletal muscles and oxygen supply to the brain, and it can suppress nerve inflammation.

Studies with rats have shown rapid increases in serotonin levels with WBV,[5] but physical measurements of brain serotonin levels can be done only in animals (as brain tissue samples must be taken). However, anecdotal evidence of increased serotonin and norepinephrine levels with WBV is strong.

> **Whole body vibration is a natural, safe, rapid, nonaddictive, and legal way to increase serotonin and norepinephrine.**

Hundreds of my clients, and thousands of users around the world, report rapid and dramatic improvements in mood, energy, and sleep within days of beginning vibration. They also report increased motivation, focus, and activity levels—perhaps the reason why Tony Robbins, the well-known motivational speaker, uses vibration machines at his seminars. Mental health benefits from WBV is an area of great potential and should be investigated more thoroughly.

Since stress and mental health are linked to chronic inflammation, WBV's capability to improve health in these areas can also help to lower inflammation.

Weight Loss: WBV can help you lose weight, which has many benefits for your health, including lowering inflammation.

Like any exercise, WBV increases your metabolism and muscle strength, both of which help you burn more calories and lose weight. Just as important, WBV raises serotonin levels; this has antidepressant effects and improves mood and sleep. Since many people overeat for emotional reasons rather than physical hunger, this effect can help in the battle to maintain and/or achieve a healthy weight. Chapter 5 focuses on how WBV helps you lose weight, the benefits to your health, and the research that supports this claim.

Hormonal Changes: Hormonal changes that come with WBV promote decreasing inflammation, weight loss, and greater energy. The stress hormone cortisol, which is elevated in chronic stress and inflammation situations, decreases.[6] This effect helps to calm the body's stress reaction and decrease belly fat, which is associated with many inflammatory conditions. Testosterone goes up, which gives both men and women greater zest and energy for life as well as increased libido; and human growth hormone (HGH) increases.[7] HGH is the major anti-aging hormone that promotes healing and repair of all tissues, including your immune system.

Pain: Chronic pain is linked to inflammation, such as with arthritis and other persistent joint and muscle pains. WBV research has shown lower pain levels in several studies looking at different types of pain in several different parts of the body[8] (see also appendix 1). Results, however, have been somewhat mixed in the area of reducing pain. I believe the issue may lie with which type of vibration machine is used and how it is used. I will discuss this issue in greater depth in chapter 4; however, many of my customers, and others, happily report precipitous drops in pain with WBV, an early and encouraging sign of decreasing inflammation.

Increasing Bone Density: Another life-changing "side effect" of WBV is increasing bone density[9]—without the toxicity and risk of bone density drugs. While the workout effect is greatest if you are exercising on your machine (chapter 13), many of the benefits, including lowering inflammation and increasing bone density, can be achieved just by standing on the vibrating plate. You can find more information about the bone density effects of WBV in my book *Whole Body Vibration for Seniors*.

Other Benefits: WBV has a profound effect on many parts of your body, including brain health, appearance, and even sexual desire—remember that increasing testosterone. For example, exercise has been shown to be the most important factor for brain health, powerfully stimulating neural cell growth and strength. Stand on a vibrating plate, and you will be stimulating muscles to contract and neurons to fire twenty to fifty times per second, which adds up to twelve to thirty thousand times in one ten-minute session—a thorough neurological stimulation. Sending signals around your body and brain is a workout for your neurons, and just as a workout strengthens your muscles, this neurological stimulation strengthens and protects your neurons.

This is a godsend for all of us—as keeping your nervous system and brain in top working order will affect every part of your life; it is especially important for people facing neurological disease and disability. You can learn more about other benefits of

WBV and the research behind these claims in my books *Whole Body Vibration: The Future of Good Health* and *Whole Body Vibration for Seniors*.

Electromagnetic Energy Effects: I believe that WBV also works on an energetic level to help guide your body and mind back to health. Evidence for this comes from the quick drop in pain levels that is often seen from just one short session of WBV—sometimes from just standing on the vibrating plate for a minute or two (see appendix 1). Such an effect could be similar to that of other vibrational energy therapies such as acupuncture, which has been shown to be remarkably effective for pain reduction.[10] For example, the Chinese sometimes perform surgery using only acupuncture as the anesthetic. In chapter 4, we will look more closely at how WBV might be affecting our electromagnetic energy system.

The Correct Type of Vibration Machine

For the best results, it is important to use the right kind of vibration machine—one that is optimized for your brain as well as for a workout. There are many types of machines—and they are not all the same. (See chapter 12 for complete explanation of machine types.)

I recommend a relatively gentle, smooth, low-stress, vertical vibration machine. This type of machine will provide your brain with a perfectly synchronized and calming vibration message.

Other types of vibration can be chaotic or too strong, delivering a garbled message to your brain and body, putting you into a fight-or-flight mode that is not conducive to healing.

TESTIMONIALS

The Vibrant Health Power 1000 is an incredible machine!!! I was skeptical at first . . . but I felt that as we are vibrational beings ourselves, there was "something" to this. I read Becky's book several times and bought the Power 1000 model because of its power and versatility. I wanted it to take me to all possible places of healing. I was suffering from chronic foot and hip pain. I noticed immediately, I'm talking after the first exposure which was only about two minutes on low, that the stabbing pain in my feet went completely away. This was eye opening for me, and I became addicted. I have watched the weight melt off relatively easily . . . which was awesome, as it had been a stubborn issue even with really healthy eating. You will notice instantly that something is happening . . . it just feels sooooo good. It's like my body said, "thank you, thank you"! Best money I ever invested in my health!!

—Lori Vandervelde, age 62

This wonderful product has been a true game-changer in my healing after a lifetime of chronic illness! I truly feel stronger every day and notice that my body is changing! So, an unexpected side effect is that I actually look younger and healthier, which is priceless!

—C. Meyers, early 50s

> I cannot make it without the Power 1000 machine! I've had it three months now—my body loves it. Increased blood flow to an aging brain helps my memory. Infection-fighting white blood cells via the lymphatic system cleanse and calm my inflamed sinus tissues and congested ears. Increased lymphatic cleansing calms my bronchial spasms. And my arthritic knees thank me every day for this purchase!
>
> —Margaret Rinicker, age 61
>
> I am excited to wake up every morning! Sleep is a joy. There is bounce in my step, and I can wear a smile out. Nothing qualifies as a chore—I find something in every activity to make it interesting.
>
> For two years before finding the Power 1000, I used another vibration machine, and followed their suggested program—without seeing benefits. I used to think all vibration was the same—not anymore!
>
> It has been a pleasure to live without the stress, weight, and shifting profile I had been coping with. Thank you, Becky, for the new body, new outlook, and new life! You have put my mind on vacation.
>
> —Doreen Fullmer, age 68

> I first heard about whole body vibration two years ago. I bought an inexpensive oscillation machine, and I increased too quickly—my body did not respond well. In 2020, when the pandemic hit, I was diagnosed with osteoarthritis and was in a lot of discomfort and pain. I began to look for solutions and bought Becky's whole body vibration machine. This machine has made all the difference. In just one week, my pain levels decreased, and my energy, strength, and mood improved. Becky Chambers's books and her work have truly been a blessing to me.
>
> —Mildred Scott, age 65
>
> I have struggled for years with chronic fatigue. The morning after my first one-minute session, I jumped out of bed for the first time in about twenty years, plus my mind is clear and focused.
>
> —Peg McNeil, 50s

Do not use a powerful double motor machine, as this type can send a desynchronizing message into your brain, potentially leading to negative mental and physical effects[11] (see chapter 12, regarding double-motor vibration machines).

For the best results, use a smooth and perfectly synchronized vibration. Ideally, you want to use a mid-level, gentle but still powerful, machine with a "purr" that is like that of a very large cat such as a cheetah. You need vibration that is strong

> *I recommend a relatively gentle, smooth, low-stress, vertical vibration machine. This type of machine will provide your brain with a perfectly synchronized and calming vibration message.*

enough to go through your entire body to achieve other effects, such as increasing bone density and getting an intense workout. If your health cannot tolerate that strong a vibration, a gentler machine of the same type can still be effective for lowering inflammation and is an excellent place to start.

Go/Start Slow: Take your time building up the speed and duration of your WBV workouts. For the best results, it is also important to use your vibration machine properly. You need vibration that is optimized for your brain as well as for a workout, and you should proceed slowly. Just as you would not try to run a marathon before you have trained for it, go slowly with your vibration machine—it will have powerful effects on your body and mind.

With WBV, doing too much too soon will sabotage your anti-inflammation plan by putting too much stress on your body—potentially leading to increasing inflammation instead of lowering it (see also chapter 9). Chapter 13 has much more information and guidelines on how to get started with a WBV program, including photos of suggested workout positions and daily WBV plans. I am also available for consultations.

To work with me, please contact me through my website: BCVibrantHealth.com.

Chapter 3

Cutting-Edge Inflammation Research

Recent research on the effects of whole body vibration on gut flora and inflammation levels in the body has triggered excitement, as there are implications for many chronic diseases.[1] These studies are providing evidence that whole body vibration improves gut flora in the digestive system and increases immune system cells that produce anti-inflammatory molecules. Beneficial changes in the gut are like knocking over the first in a row of dominos, as gut health is one of the major origins of inflammation (see chapter 8). Gut inflammatory diseases will be alleviated by these changes, but the results also may

Whole body vibration improves gut flora in the digestive system and increases immune system cells that produce anti-inflammatory molecules.

have implications for diabetes and obesity,[2] as well as other serious diseases driven by inflammation.

Gut Flora Changes with Whole Body Vibration

Research with mice at the Medical College of Georgia in 2019[3] showed a seventeen-fold increase in the gut bacteria *Alistipes*—a gut bacteria that plays a key role in reducing inflammation in the gut. *Alistipes* is a prolific producer of short-chain fatty acids which decrease gut inflammation. In the words of Dr. Jack Yu, lead researcher in this groundbreaking study, "these bacteria are very good at decreasing inflammation in the gut."[4]

Whole body vibration (WBV) also led to a marked increase in M2 macrophages, a type of immune system cell which suppresses or halts inflammation. In a positive feedback loop, the increase in *Alistipes* leads to an increase in M2 macrophages, which produce natural anti-inflammatory molecules called cytokines, such as interleukin-10.

Alistipes also help ferment food in the gut properly, improving metabolism and enhancing the availability of glucose for human usage (vs. detrimental gut flora) in the gastrointestinal tract. Another metabolic benefit of *Alistipes* is that butyrate, one of the short-chain fatty acids that this bacteria produces, can help reverse the negative effects of a high-fat diet. These 2019 results confirm previous research showing improved blood sugar control and insulin resistance with WBV.[5]

> **Whole body vibration also led to a marked increase in M2 macrophages, a type of immune system cell which suppresses or halts inflammation.**

Another study showed increases in the level of beneficial *Lactobacillus* bacteria in mice and people after vibration.[6] *Lactobacillus* bacteria have been associated with good intestinal health.[7] This finding is why *Lactobacillus* is one of the major types of bacteria in the probiotic products so commonly advertised on TV, radio, and the Internet. These products are effective for reducing digestive system symptoms because they can help restore proper gut flora balance, which reduces inflammation.

While the improvements to gut health are clear, exactly how WBV effects changes in our gut bacteria and inflammation factors has not yet been determined, but it appears that the effect is real. As Dr Jack Yu, author of the 2019 Medical College of Georgia research, puts it, "The sequencing is not yet completely clear, but it appears to be a closed-loop, feed forward, self-magnifying cycle."[8]

Emotional stress is well known to increase inflammation and be linked to poor health. I believe that the same energetic effect that may lie behind decreases in pain with WBV, might also explain how "an activity that mimics exercise without any of the active movement can have such a positive chain reaction."[9] Our thoughts and emotions create energy—an energy that can be measured with an MRI of our brain—and every emotion is linked to a chemical reaction in our body. As our energetic system is inextricably linked to our mind, body, and nervous system, to achieve the best results in reducing inflammation, it is important to use the best type of vibration for the brain and nervous system. Several of the studies discussed above report using vertical vibration. Vertical vibration produces less stress due to its smooth, calm motion—potentially a key element in reducing inflammation.

> **Studies with people using WBV have shown groundbreaking changes in cytokines, interleukins, and other molecules that the immune system uses to regulate the inflammatory response, as well as stem cells and other factors that promote healing.**

Research on Inflammation Markers, Cytokines, and Stem Cells

Studies with people using WBV have shown groundbreaking changes in cytokines, interleukins, and other molecules that the immune system uses to regulate the inflammatory response, as well as stem cells and other factors that promote healing. These molecules circulate in the bloodstream with implications for many diseases, particularly heart disease, blood pressure, diabetes, wound healing, and decreased inflammation throughout the body. One closely studied anti-inflammatory cytokine, interleukin-10 (IL-10), helps to calm the immune system, while another interleukin (IL-6) increases inflammation.

For repair and regeneration of the body, stem cells are the holy grail. These cells are unique in their ability to develop into many different types of cells and thus regenerate tissues and organs all over the body. They have the potential to become

---

TESTIMONIALS

Becky Chambers combines vast knowledge and experience with two powerful energy medicines in her book Homeopathy Plus Whole Body Vibration. **In this case, the whole is far greater than the sum of the parts. In just a couple of weeks with the help of a homeopathic remedy, whole body vibration, changing my diet, and getting rid of** Candida **yeast (restoring balance to gut flora), I actually woke up feeling great, and three inches were off my waist too! Over the next four months, with the help of more homeopathics and continued WBV, I've lost a total of forty-five previously very stubborn pounds and five inches off my waist, and my mood and energy are better than ever.**

—*Dr. D. L. Camhi, chiropractor, age 60*

> I am super pleased with my purchase of Becky's Vibrant Health Power 1000. Having been aware of these types of machines for years, I was convinced of the well-documented benefits, and was ready and eager to purchase—but so confused by the choices!! Wisely, I read Becky's book on whole body vibration. I phoned her with additional questions about what the right choice for me would be, personally, and ordered the Power 1000. I have used it every day for the last six months and will continue to use it every day to come. I have various autoimmune conditions, including rheumatoid arthritis. I can't quite explain the mechanism of action it has on my body, I just know I feel a whole lot better. When I'm up for it, I incorporate the exercises and positions suggested on the accompanying WBV poster, and that really makes a difference. You can really step up your routine when you want. It feels good just to stand—or sit—on it, too. Effective either way. I always get a lift when I need it, and when I'm looking for calming and relaxation, this somehow helps with that, too.
>
> —Cathy Hlywak, mid-50s

specialized cells as varied as muscle cells, blood cells, and brain cells. Also carefully tracked are other regenerative molecules that increase angiogenesis, the development and repair of blood vessels. Drug companies have been working for years to achieve beneficial changes with these healing factors. It appears that you can gain these anti-inflammatory and regenerative changes, and with greater safety and ease, just by standing on your vibration machine.

An exciting study by the US military, released in 2020, compared the anti-inflammation and regenerative healing effects of WBV to that of standard exercise and found WBV to be superior in several important areas. Inflammation marker levels for IL-10 and IL-6, and two angiogenesis factors,[iii] improved significantly with WBV; lesser effects were seen with either exercise alone or exercise and WBV.[10]

Inflammation marker levels for IL-10 and IL-6, and two angiogenesis factors, improved significantly with WBV; lesser effects were seen with either exercise alone or exercise and WBV.

In addition, the highest levels of stem cells and other regenerative growth factors were seen with the use of WBV plus exercise. WBV plus exercise led to a 39 percent increase in angiogenic circulating stem cells, a 33 percent increase with WBV alone, and a 21 percent increase with exercise only.

This study was split into a younger group of subjects (average age 24) and an older group (average age 55). Not surprisingly, the best results across the board were seen in the younger group, but the older group showed similar improvements for levels of

---

[iii]Tumor necrosis factor alpha (TNF) and vascular endothelial growth factor (VEGF)—two molecules your body produces that promote the growth of new blood vessels.

anti-inflammatory markers and not quite as good but still significant improvements in stem cell levels. The study's conclusion: WBV "may offer a viable treatment option to help attenuate inflammation and increase stem/progenitor cell circulation."[11]

WBV plus exercise led to a 39 percent increase in angiogenic circulating stem cells, a 33 percent increase with WBV alone, and a 21 percent increase with exercise only.

These inflammation lowering results confirm earlier studies. A study in 2015, with healthy elderly people, showed a drop in C-reactive protein and other inflammatory system regulatory markers called "toll-like receptors."[12] C-reactive protein (CRP) is made by your liver and is a good bellwether for inflammation. Toll-like receptors help the immune system to quickly recognize pathogens and turn up inflammation levels. Thus, dropping levels of CRP and toll-like receptors are a sign that inflammation is also dropping. Another study, in 2012, with elderly people with knee osteoarthritis, also found that pain and inflammatory cytokine levels dropped.[13] Similar anti-inflammatory results were found in a 2017 study looking at WBV and fibromyalgia.[14]

However, while these results are exciting, it has not been easy to replicate them in older people with significant health issues. In fact, a systematic review in 2015 of five research studies on WBV for people with knee arthritis,[15] only two of these five studies, all of which were on people age sixty to seventy-five, were able to show a reduction in inflammation and/or pain. Also, a number of the other studies reporting good results were done with younger subjects, such as the military study and the fibromyalgia study—and younger people typically have a greater ability to heal and respond well to interventions.

Also keep in mind that most of these studies do not use the type of vibration I recommend, or, when they occasionally do, they do not follow the protocol I recommend, nor do they combine WBV with the other methods in this book to reduce inflammation. With an approach combining all these elements, it is possible that you may get better results.

Important: In my twenty years of experience with WBV, I have seen that gentler machines, carefully designed for both the mind and the body, lead to better results, especially combined with a slower, more gradual buildup in the amount of vibration and the addition of other positive health methods as outlined in this book.

Many of the research studies are done using the type of machine that was originally developed for use with Olympic athletes—a powerful, double motor, tri-planar vibration machine. (See chapter 12 for more information about different types of vibration machines.) This is a type of machine that I don't recommend, especially for older people and those with health issues, because it is too powerful and desynchronizing for the nervous system and mind. From my experience and research, achieving significant anti-inflammatory and regenerative healing results with older people who have health issues requires a gentler, completely synchronized type of vibration. And combining WBV

TESTIMONIALS

I bought a machine from Becky two years ago. I have more muscle mass and virtually no pain now. I had pain before if my spine was out of alignment for more than a minute or two—like in a new car seat! I still try to stay in alignment, but if I am forced to sit in an uncomfortable seat for a while, it no longer cripples me. WBV also helps my energy level; if I am tired, it revives me more than coffee would. I am so glad I bought this machine. I am seventy-one years old, teach yoga, and am amazing myself and my doctor with the results this machine has given me.

—Jacqueline Farless, age 71

My husband and I both use this machine and love it. I am a nurse who works twelve-hour shifts, and at the end of my shift, my feet and lower legs are really aching. I also have had a lot of pain in my shoulder and neck at the end of my shifts. We have been using the machine now for about a year and a half, and it has greatly helped both of us. I use it in the morning, and also before going to bed—then I am able to go right to sleep without moving my legs a lot trying to get them to stop hurting enough to go to sleep. I also have not had any more neck or shoulder pain since using the machine. Plus, WBV has given my husband and I more endurance.

—C. Seaton, late 50s

with other important aspects of health care, such as a targeted diet and exercise program, only makes sense.

WBV for Obesity-Related Inflammation

Obesity can lead to chronic inflammation, which can trigger other diseases such as atherosclerosis (the most common form of cardiovascular disease), type 2 diabetes, and even cancer. Weight gain and obesity are major health risks and have a long list of associated diseases; nonetheless, as steadily increasing rates of obesity and weight gain over the past century make clear, it is a difficult issue to turn around. This makes WBV's capacity to help people reduce weight (see chapter 5) and the health risks associated with obesity-linked inflammation one of its most valuable gifts.

One session of WBV training showed improved inflammation and metabolic responses that could lead to decreased plaque formation and lower risk of diabetes.

Obesity is a risk factor for atherosclerosis, a disease of the arteries where "plaques" of fatty material are deposited on their inner walls. As the arteries become more blocked, symptoms develop; if they become fully blocked, it can lead to strokes, heart attacks, and death. Plaques begin, however, with an inflammatory immune system process that results in lipid- (fat) rich "foam" cells in the blood, which eventually create plaques. It is well known that one of the most effective methods for preventing both obesity and atherosclerosis is regular exercise.[16]

A 2020 study with obese and normal weight people (21 men and women, 18–45 years of age) engaging in one session of WBV training showed improved inflammation and metabolic responses that could lead to decreased plaque formation and lower risk of diabetes.[17] This study found that the anti-inflammatory effects of IL-6 (which modulates the inflammatory reaction and thus can be either pro-inflammatory or anti-inflammatory, depending on the circumstances) increased with WBV and that there were

> **TESTIMONIAL**
>
> **I am thrilled with my vibration machine. Combining vibration with diet changes and a *Candida* yeast program, I have lost forty pounds in six months—after many years of trying to lose weight with little success. My legs are no longer swollen, and I am off my diuretic medication. I also have had high cholesterol my entire adult life (everybody in my family has high cholesterol), and I have been on Lipitor for years. My cholesterol has now dropped eighty points, and I am off Lipitor. My triglycerides were very high (332)—they have dropped over a hundred points to 214. My gas, bloating, and heartburn have disappeared, and my face is clear—the puffiness, poor color, and minor acne is gone.**
>
> —Angelica, age 57

corresponding improvements in glucose metabolism, reducing the risk of both diabetes and heart disease. The results of this study showed that a single session of WBV had similar metabolic and immune system effects as a single session of traditional exercise for both obese and normal weight people.

Chapter 4

Whole Body Vibration and Pain

When there are nerves in the area of inflammation, there will also be pain. As a 2021 scientific review of pain management noted, "pain is a consequential phenomenon of inflammatory responses."[1] With pain being a major quality of life factor for millions of people, and dependence on pain killing drugs leading to further health issues and possibly more inflammation,[2] the capacity to reduce pain is a life-changing benefit of WBV.

There is research that has shown evidence that some types of pain, such as chronic lower back pain,[3] muscle pain,[4] fibromyalgia,[5] and knee pain from osteoarthritis,[6] decrease with WBV. But in other research for some types of pain—for example, knee osteoarthritis—the results have not been clear. While some studies with older people conclude that WBV improves knee osteoarthritis pain,[7] others conclude that it doesn't.[8] In the same systematic review of WBV's effects on knee arthritis mentioned earlier,[9] the combined data showed statistically

> **With pain being a major quality of life factor for millions of people, and dependence on pain killing drugs leading to further health issues and possibly more inflammation, the capacity to reduce pain is a life-changing benefit of WBV.**

significant improvement in knee pain and function. But, individually, only two of the five studies in that meta-analysis concluded that knee pain was reduced.[10] Another systematic review concluded that knee osteoarthritis pain does not decrease with WBV.[11]

What accounts for the conflicting results? The answer is similar to the issue regarding reducing inflammation with WBV. Success may lie in how and what type of WBV is used, especially with more fragile populations, such as older people and those with health issues.

When the correct type of vibration is used, and my guidelines for a slow and gentle approach are followed, I have had clear positive results for pain reduction in older people. While not every person in my survey reported a reduction in pain, *some people reported nearly complete disappearances of pain within weeks of beginning WBV, and for all those in pain, the overall average pain reduction was 31 percent* (see appendix 1). This survey covered many different types and locations of pain—back pain, joint pain, muscle pain, and nerve pain. As mentioned earlier, these results also included some people who reduced their pain medication at the same time.

Many of these people were also using other natural health methods in addition to WBV, but as they had usually been using those methods for years before adding WBV to their regimen, it seems that WBV was the trigger for their sudden improvements. I do, however, recommend adding other natural health methods to your WBV program, because they can work synergistically, leading to greater effects.

Possibly WBV may even be of use in the fight against opioid addiction, in particular by helping people to avoid becoming addicted in the first place. While WBV is not recommended for immediate use after acute injuries or procedures and cannot replace powerful opioids, WBV is an effective natural system to lower pain without the use of drugs.

While not every person in my survey reported a reduction in pain, some people reported nearly complete disappearances of pain within weeks of beginning WBV, and for all those in pain, the overall average pain reduction was 31 percent.

WBV also raises serotonin, norepinephrine, and testosterone, which can give people the boost to mood and energy that they often seek from opioids.

With the aid of these effects, WBV may be of help in weaning people off, or possibly avoiding entirely, addictive pain killers for chronic conditions, thus avoiding addiction. For example, in my research survey (appendix 1) 74 percent of those in pain reported a 50 percent drop in pain, and some of those people reported that they were also reducing the amount of their pain medication or switching to less powerful pain medication.

How Does Whole Body Vibration Relieve Pain?

My recommendations, which seem to lead to greater success for pain relief than other methods, are to start with only one minute at the lowest speed setting on one of my machines; then, very gradually build up, adding one minute to your daily vibration every two to five days while staying at the lowest speed. You do not have to perform exercises on the machine to see these reductions in pain—just stand or sit on the vibrating plate. This is not a significant workout, but, in fact, every muscle and cell is being stimulated and invigorated by the vibration as it travels from your feet up through your body, causing a cascade of benefits: increased blood flow—supplying nutrients and oxygen and removing waste products—and nervous system activation. With the right kind of vibration, you will immediately feel this enlivening effect from head to toe.

Electromagnetic Energy

I also believe that there may be an effect of vibration on the body's electromagnetic energy; perhaps in a manner similar to numerous other forms of "energy medicine," such as acupuncture, tai chi, and homeopathy, which are known for their ability to decrease pain.[12] Western medicine recognizes that the nervous system is a pattern of electromagnetic signals—an electroencephalogram (EEG) measures the electrical activity of the brain, and magnetic resonance imaging (MRI) creates images of the brain by measuring its electromagnetic energy.

Dr. Norm Shealy, one of the early advocates of alternative health and an innovator in energy and pain medicine, reports marked improvement—using acupuncture only—in 70 percent of people with rheumatoid arthritis who failed to improve with conventional medicine; 75 percent of people with migraines; 80 percent of people with diabetic neuropathy; 70 percent of people with depression; and 70 percent of people with chronic low back pain.[13]

Many cultures throughout time have recognized the existence of a life-force energy. The Chinese call it chi, Indians call it prana, and European traditions have called it variously life force, soul, spirit, vital energy, vital principle, elan, and more. This energy guides and powers one's body and life, and disturbances in this energy due to trauma of any sort can have a profound effect on your physical and mental state.

Thousands of years ago, the Chinese discovered and mapped "energy meridians" in the body. Each of these energy pathways is associated with different organs and bodily systems. The Chinese medical system of acupuncture is based on maintaining a healthy and balanced flow of energy in those different meridians. Indian medicine describes chakras, spinning energy vortexes in our bodies, also associated with particular body systems and organs. In fact, some people can sense their own vibrational energy, and when these people stand on a vibrating plate, they report feeling energy shooting through their energy meridians and their chakras unblocking and spinning faster.

There is, in fact, measurable electromagnetic energy emanating from all things, because all substances are made from molecules that are, in turn, made from even smaller vibrating particles that have positive or negative electrical charges. Thus, every substance has an electromagnetic charge that can be measured with sensitive scientific equipment. For example, Kirlian photography can detect and record the electromagnetic wavelengths around a person or object.[14]

Electrodermal Testing

Another energy-measuring system that is frequently used by medical doctors in Europe, where it was first developed in the 1950s, is called "electrodermal testing." This is a computer-linked testing system in which a probe that detects electromagnetic energy is touched to different acupuncture points on the hands and feet, and the energy in the associated meridian is graphed out on the computer screen.[15] With this system, one can instantly see which energy meridians, thus their associated body organs or systems, are in balance, stressed (too much energy), or weakened (too little energy).

There are more than one hundred thousand such electrodermal screening machines in use worldwide, though very few are in the US, where acceptance of energy medicine has been limited. There are many accounts of the detection of diseases, allergies, and toxic states using these machines.[16] One can also see, before spending a lot of time and money, which therapies or products resonate with an individual's electromagnetic energy and are therefore most likely to be successful. Electrodermal testing will also register changes in energy before and after vibration, as I have seen in my natural health practice, where I have used both vibration and electrodermal testing.

Piezoelectricity

Theoretically, WBV could affect our energy meridians in a similar manner to acupuncture through the property of piezoelectricity. Piezoelectricity is the ability of crystals to turn mechanical vibration into electrical vibration. Our bodies can be thought of as living liquid crystals, in the sense that we are highly organized molecular structures, and, as such, we would have the property of piezoelectricity. Shealy thus describes our "bodies, souls, minds, and emotional realm" as a "living matrix"[17] with the property of piezoelectricity: "Waves of mechanical vibration moving through the living matrix produce electrical fields and vice versa. . . . Connective tissue is a liquid crystalline semiconductor. Piezoelectric signals from the cells can travel throughout the body in this medium."[18] The result is that "energetic treatment of one part of this living matrix always affects the whole."[19]

Thus, in theory, every time you are on a vibration plate and your neurons fire, shooting electromagnetic energy through your body and brain, your body could be turning the mechanical vibration into the electrical energy vibrations you need to heal, balance, and unblock your energy systems. Energy would then flow into and through your energy meridians and chakra energy centers, increasing their proper spinning and energy flow. As these energy meridians and chakras are also linked (in

Chinese medicine) to different organs, body systems, emotions, and needs, improving the flow of energy could help heal the physical body and mind and improve life—all at the same time.

I have seen hundreds of people step on a whole body vibration plate only to get off one to two minutes later with their pain gone. I want to keep an open mind as to how this might be happening. The placebo effect is unlikely, as this often happens with people who have never heard of the possibility. For example, at crowded expos where I don't have time to mention it to people who have never even heard of WBV before.

More research needs to be done to determine exactly how vibration can create such quick and powerful reductions in pain, but perhaps WBV could be similar to acupuncture in its ability to stimulate our electromagnetic system.

> ## TESTIMONIALS
>
> **When I first started working with Becky, about three months ago, I had constant pain in my right hip, right thigh, and both knees. I frequently walked with a limp, and climbing stairs was excruciatingly painful. In the last three months, I have made dramatic improvements. I was able to return to moderate exercising, and I have no pain in my hips or thighs. If anyone had told me that I could be so much stronger or that my pain could be reduced so much in such a brief period of time, I never would have believed it.**
>
> —Ann MacGibbon, PhD, age 50s

> **Three days after receiving my vibration machine:** Becky—you won't believe this! I have been on the WBV plate three days, now up to two minutes per day. My hip pain had been waking me up during the night for months. Well, yesterday I walked a couple of miles (which usually aggravates my hip). Last night—no pain!! and only a little today. Wow. Amazing!!!!!!!!!!!! Thank you bunches—can't wait to work up to ten minutes and the exercises.
>
> *Update after three months of vibration:* I originally got my vibration machine because my eye doctor suggested it as a way to help my hip and bone density. It is too soon to know about those issues, but recently I had an eye pressure test for glaucoma, three months after starting vibration. Last year, I was at risk of glaucoma with eye pressure readings nearing a diagnosable level. This year, my readings are down to where I am not considered at risk anymore. The only thing I've changed is adding WBV and extra vitamins for my eyes. My eye doctor thinks it is the combination of the two that has helped my eyes! Thank you!
>
> —Connie W., age 64

In 2008, according to the medical profession, I needed both shoulders replaced. I was in a great deal of pain for years and was unable to raise my arms to reach anything above my head due to the pain and joint limitations. I had to modify all my exercise and drop cross-country skiing, mountain climbing, and yoga because of the pain and limited use of my shoulders and upper body. Depression from this limiting situation had me crying many days, as exercise and wellness had always been a huge part of my life. The pain was intense, twenty-four hours a day.

After only a few sessions, starting at only one minute the first time and increasing only one minute per session, I noticed I was starting to feel better. At first, I wouldn't tell anyone, because I couldn't believe it! But I continued to improve.

Vibrating, in combination with eating well and an exercise program, has been a huge factor in lessening the twenty-four-hour pain I had in both shoulders. The shoulders still need replacing, but, because the pain is not bothering me, I can postpone the medical procedure.

—Wendy MacLean, small business co-owner, senior citizen

Chapter 5

Losing Weight with Whole Body Vibration

When it comes to lowering inflammation, weight loss is an elephant stuck in the room—hard to move and impossible to ignore; critical to get help with! One of the most exciting aspects of whole body vibration (WBV) for many people, and especially for people battling inflammation and chronic health issues, is that WBV can help you lose weight. As one of the most hotly researched topics, the evidence is clear: adding whole body vibration to a program of healthy eating and exercise expedites weight loss.

Whole body vibration can help you lose weight and keep it off long term by speeding up your metabolism, balancing gut flora, increasing energy levels, elevating your mood, and strengthening muscles—all with a short ten to fifteen minute daily routine of vibration exercise. My own research and experience show that even if all you do is stand on the plate, you are still getting many benefits, including help losing weight. Now

Whole body vibration can help you lose weight and keep it off long term by speeding up your metabolism, balancing gut flora, increasing energy levels, elevating your mood, and strengthening muscles—all with a short ten to fifteen minute daily routine of vibration exercise.

you might be laughing, but don't let the laughter stop you.

A 2018 systematic review[1] of eighteen research articles, with a combined total of 321 human subjects, looked at using WBV with obese patients. The results showed increased metabolism and weight and fat loss, along with improvements in other issues known to be related to obesity, such as heart health, peripheral and central circulation, glucose regulation, and inflammation levels. Increased weight loss with WBV was confirmed again in 2019 with another large systematic review of thirteen clinical trials on the subject.[2]

My own research, and my extensive experience with clients and myself, also make it clear that WBV is a huge plus in any weight-loss program. In Vibrant Health's 2019 survey of our customers, 50 percent of those who wanted to lose weight reported that they did indeed lose weight.[3] This is a high success rate in an area where success rates are usually low. Our research is in line with other research showing modest but long-term weight loss with WBV, especially when combined with diet and exercise.

How Whole Body Vibration Helps You Lose Weight

- WBV can be an intense workout, and, like any workout, this will increase your metabolic rate so that you burn more calories and lose weight more easily—and the time required to achieve the same results as with traditional exercise forms is much less. In fact, with a powerful vibration machine, ten to fifteen minutes of WBV equals one hour of conventional weight training. Anyone who tries working out on a WBV machine will see the truth of this effect, and mathematical calculations of the force exerted based on mass, acceleration, and gravitation prove the point. See chapter 13 for more on how to exercise with WBV.

- The workout builds lean muscle mass that will continue to burn more calories all day. First, a workout triggers the growth of muscle tissue through protein synthesis, one of the highest energy or calorie burning activities for our cells. Then, all day long, muscle tissue is metabolically more active and burns calories faster than fat cells. Lean muscle mass can account for 60 percent of your energy and calorie expenditure while at rest.

- WBV raises serotonin levels in your brain,[4] which has a powerful antidepressant effect that will help you eat properly and be more active. Everybody knows they should eat well (and probably smaller quantities) and exercise more to lose weight; the problem is actually doing it. WBV helps you to be in that calm and relaxed but energized mental state in which you can focus and achieve your goals.

- WBV balances gut flora, which can help you lose weight. Gut bacteria have roles in digestion, fat storage, hunger, mood, and food cravings, all of which can have major impacts on your weight. Balancing gut flora also calms gut inflammation, which leads to a drop in water retention and bloating that can give you quick improvements on the scale.

- WBV gives you strength (increased muscle power) and energy. So when you do exercise, now more often because your energy is up and you are in a better mood, you will work harder, consequently burning more calories.
- WBV lowers cortisol levels.[5] Cortisol is a major stress and aging hormone that promotes fat production and storage. Lowering cortisol levels helps promote fat burning and proper fat metabolism.
- WBV improves joint health and lowers pain in numerous ways so that you have greater mobility.[6] Along with increased energy and a better mood, this leads to more activity.

TESTIMONIALS

I feel like I have always been trying to lose weight. ... Then, two years ago, my daughter came home from college and said she was going to lose some weight over the summer. I decided to join her. To my utter dismay, I weighed in at 178 lbs! Way too much for my 5'2" petite frame. At first, I struggled to lose any weight. After reading Becky's book, I purchased the Power 1000 vibration machine and began to lose some weight. But then, right before Covid hit, I fell and broke my arm, then came Covid, and I lost my job after twenty-four years with the company. My father died a month later, and I realized this was a lot of traumas all at once. I decided to look at the time off as a blessing and focused on taking care of myself.

I got serious. . . . I went to see a functional medicine doctor who helped balance my hormones, I ate a very clean diet and exercised every day, and I vibrated every day for fifteen minutes and incorporated a dry sauna into my routine. I am happy to report, two years later, that I now weigh 128 lbs—a loss of 50 lbs! My daughter says I am aging backwards!

I really believe the Power 1000 was instrumental in helping me lose weight and keep it off, and a side benefit of vibrating every day is that the pain in my feet and ankles that I was plagued with for years is gone. I noticed that the pain was gone around two months after I started using my machine daily—I was out walking with my son and he asked me how my foot pain was, and I realized it was gone, TOTALLY!

Thank you, Becky for your dedication; you have really helped turn my life around. I am so looking forward to your next book!

—Sandy O'Brien, age 58

I've been using WBV and working with Becky for about fifteen years. When I first started, I was forty-seven years old, and I lost thirty pounds in six months. I felt like the Energizer Bunny: I was full of energy, my hay fever and headaches went away, my mood improved, and I became much stronger than I had ever been.

Then I moved out of state, fell out of touch, and stopped using vibration. Gradually, I gained all the weight back plus more, and my health issues came back. Six years later, I returned and began working with Becky again. The weight is coming off more slowly this time, but I have lost about twenty pounds so far, and as long as I eat well, and vibrate, I can lose weight again.

Mostly, thank God for Becky's incredible ability to help me with my health issues! Over the years, with the help of WBV and Becky's "magic" homeopathic remedies, she has helped me with so many debilitating health issues: joint pain, weakness, dizziness, nausea, headaches, skin rashes, hot flashes and night sweats, fatigue, wheezing, anxiety, depression, and grief after the deaths of multiple family members and friends.

Today, I am proud to say, I am strong and healthy, working and enjoying my life, calmer and more balanced than ever. Thank you, Becky.

—Doreen Hadge, age 62

Scientific Research

The early research with animals was very exciting. In a 2007 study of mice that received fifteen minutes of daily vibration for twelve weeks, the mice that got vibration ended up with 27 percent lower amounts of fat, along with corresponding increases in bone density, than the control mice that didn't get any vibration.[7] In the photo from this study, the dark areas are fat, and the mice who received vibration are visibly considerably leaner and have less of the dark fat areas.

By 2020, there had been many research studies using humans as subjects, and the results were less dramatic than they had been with mice but still encouraging. With mice, their diet and other activities could be controlled but not so with human subjects. The mice used in studies are also young mice, and younger animals (human

> *Mice that got vibration ended up with 27 percent lower amounts of fat, along with corresponding increases in bone density, than the control mice that didn't get any vibration.*

Mice Exposed to Vibration

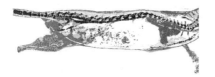

Normal Mice

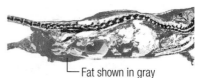

Fat shown in gray

Source: Clinton Rubin; PNAS. Used by permission of Dr. Clinton Rubin, the *New York Times*.

or mouse) have a greater regenerative ability and can tolerate physical stress more easily, which can lead to better results. In the large 2018 systematic-review meta-analysis mentioned at the beginning of this chapter, a total of eighteen high-quality research studies and 321 subjects were included.[8] The combined results of these studies led to the conclusion that "six to twelve weeks of WBVT [Whole Body Vibration Training] in obese individuals generally led to a reduction in fat mass and cardiovascular improvements."[9]

Eight studies in the review reported a body weight decrease from 5 to 10 percent,[10] with one twenty-four-week study showing continued weight loss. That long-term study, of sixty-one overweight and obese adults, saw significant weight loss with a combination of WBV and diet, with the best long-term results obtained for those participants who combined WBV with aerobic exercise and diet. Their conclusions were that

> combining either aerobic exercise or WBV training with caloric restrictions can help to achieve a sustained long-term weight loss of 5–10%. WBV training may have the potential to reduce VAT [visceral adipose tissue; i.e., fat] more than aerobic exercise in obese adults. . . . Only Fitness and Vibration (partic-

ipants) managed to maintain a weight loss of 5% or more in the long term.[11]

Fat mass reductions of 2 to 6 percent were seen in seven of the studies[12] in that same 2018 review, including in some of the studies where there was no weight change reported. The weight loss was due to a loss of fat, not lean muscle mass; no studies reported a loss in lean muscle mass. One study reported an increase in lean muscle mass.[13] Leg muscle strength improved by 8 to 18 percent in four of the eighteen studies.

Twelve of the eighteen studies also looked at arterial and cardiovascular health. Ten studies reported improvements in various measurements of arterial stiffness, with five studies reporting large decreases in blood pressure.[14] One study[15] reported a reduction in LDL cholesterol and triglyceride concentrations in the blood.

Additional benefits found included a decline in falling incidences,[16] an increase in oxygen uptake,[17] and an increase in resting energy expenditure,[18] meaning one would be burning fat more efficiently all day.

Hormone Changes

In 2017, there was great excitement when Meghan McGee-Lawrence, a researcher at the Medical College of Georgia in Augusta, showed that metabolic and inflammation markers were significantly reduced in type 2 diabetic mice from WBV.[19] McGee's results confirmed similar results in an earlier study.[20] *Science* magazine, one of the most highly respected scientific journals in the country, greeted the new research with a hopeful article reporting that "whole-body vibration provides similar metabolic benefits as walking on a treadmill, suggesting it may be useful for treating obesity and Type II diabetes."[21] These beneficial changes in glucose metabolism and insulin resistance were confirmed in the 2019 study showing the dramatic changes in gut flora and inflammation discussed in chapter 3.[22]

Similar effects were seen in 2014 in one of the studies later included in the 2018 review discussed earlier. That study reported a large decrease in fasting insulin levels, which is an indication of improving insulin and glucose metabolism, lowering the risk of insulin resistance, prediabetic and diabetic conditions, high blood sugar levels, and hyperglycemia.[23] Leptin levels and adiponectin levels also became more balanced. Leptin levels, which are involved in appetite regulation and thermogenesis (heat production) and are typically elevated in obese people, decreased. Adiponectin, another hormone that helps control glucose regulation and fatty acid oxidation and is generally depressed in obese patients, increased.

Start Slow

Most research on weight loss with WBV puts a lot of emphasis on the exercise effect. Virtually all the studies in the 2018 review had participants performing a series of exercises while vibrating, often on very powerful vibration machines. While exercise is an essential part of health and long-term weight control, my experience and research indicate that for people with health issues, it is better to begin a WBV program with a small amount of vibration on a more modulated vibration machine and build up slowly; it is not necessary to be exercising on the vibration plate, especially at the beginning.

I believe that a slow start yields better results because WBV has so many powerful effects that can potentially increase inflammation with excessive use, including a potent detoxification effect that will further stress already stressed detoxification systems and organs. As the goal is to lower stress and thus inflammation, not just to burn calories, starting out too fast and using too powerful a machine could have the opposite effect.

When you are in pain, exhausted, or unmotivated, it is fine to simply stand on the plate. The vibration will flow through your body and mind, helping to reduce your pain and inflammation,

> ## Testimonial
>
> **Becky's machine is amazing!!! Having this machine in a place in my home with easy access and a great view made all the difference in developing my vibration routine. These machines are life changing! Aches and pain all but disappeared, and mood and weight changes happened within days! I feel better inside and out! People ask, what are you doing different? . . . BEST money ever spent!!!!I love this machine! I am so happy I got it!**
>
> **—Polly Gugino, age 61**

improve mood and focus, and improve energy and strength. When you feel better, it will be easy to add in a more rigorous exercise plan. In Vibrant Health's 2019 survey of our customers, 64 percent of the respondents reported that they followed my recommendation to start slowly, and 54 percent said that this was important for their success.[24]

Theresa Wright participated in a WBV class with the author. The class met once a week for six weeks. Each participant was given one minute of vibration during the first session, and each succeeding week the amount was increased by one minute (the class was held only once per week, which means she received a total of one minute of WBV the first week, two minutes the second week, etc.). Participants began to use exercise positions in the third week. For the first two weeks, they only stood on the plate.

> ## TESTIMONIAL
>
> **I experienced an immediate response to my first whole body vibration session. In the first class, we were each allowed one minute of WBV. Standing on the machine, I felt a powerful soothing sensation in my body. Following the first class, I also felt more energetic. Within two days, I felt more relaxed than before, handled stress better, and my energy level was growing.**
>
> **Five days after the first session, I experienced a day of super high energy, something I haven't felt for many years. This was the energy level I had had most of my life but that had been gone**

> for several years. Great stamina was back, and cleaning chores were enjoyable and easy. Spending long hours at the computer at my last job before I retired left me hating to use my home computer. Now suddenly that disappeared, and I once again enjoyed using the computer. I couldn't believe how dramatically I was responding to the WBV.
>
> Then there is the weight issue. By combining a healthy diet, natural supplements, exercise, and whole body vibration, I lost nine pounds in six weeks. Having tried to lose weight many times without success, I am sure the whole body vibration helped make the difference. My scale has blessed me with a number I haven't seen in years.
>
> —Teresa Wright, early 60s

Vibrant Health's Research

Regarding weight loss, our 2019 Vibrant Health survey results (appendix 1) are similar to the published research discussed above. In our survey of Vibrant Health customers, 50 percent of those who wanted to lose weight did lose, with 24 percent of this group losing one to ten pounds, 10 percent losing ten to twenty pounds, 5 percent losing twenty to thirty pounds, and 10 percent losing more than thirty pounds.[25] Most of our customers (90%) are over age fifty, which makes this weight loss more impressive, as it gets harder to lose weight as you get older. Since our customers were mostly not obese, just mildly to moderately overweight, the amount of weight lost is quite significant. An average weight loss of about fifteen pounds, for an estimated average weight person of 150 pounds, would be a 10 percent weight loss; and as this survey covered two years, this weight loss was well maintained.

Troubleshooting

While I have seen excellent results with many clients (and myself: I once weighed two hundred pounds but now at 5'6", I have been 120–125 pounds for many years), there can be other issues that need to be addressed. If you are not losing weight and inches while using WBV, aerobically exercising, and eating a healthy, low-carb diet, possible reasons include:

In my research survey of people using Vibrant Health machines, 50 percent of those who wanted to lose weight did lose, sometimes more than thirty pounds.

1. **Too much vibration too soon:** Vibration has powerful effects on every part of your body, stimulating every system to work harder, so it can be stressful for you, even while helping you heal and achieve greater health. Too much vibration too soon can stress your body, leading to a temporary increase in inflammation that can cause any health issue to worsen, possibly causing water retention and difficulty losing weight.

Though it is hard to believe, one thing to try if you are not seeing weight loss is to vibrate less. Everybody wants to vibrate more, thinking more exercise will help. But in this case, because the total effect of WBV is so great, less is more. Many of my clients do best starting with one minute and increasing slowly.

2. Gut Flora Imbalance: A common issue is an imbalance of the microorganisms within our intestines.[26] These microorganisms consist of various strains of bacteria, fungi, and protozoa. Collectively, these microorganisms are known as gut flora. They are essential for digestion and immune functioning, but when the balance is upset, it can result in inflammation leading to many digestive and other systemic health issues, including numerous digestive symptoms, weight gain, bloating, and water retention.

Used properly, WBV will help to balance the gut flora, and this can lead to quick weight loss as inflammation and associated water retention drains away. Conversely, because WBV is also a powerful detoxification system, too much WBV can put a strain on detoxification organs such as your liver, which can temporarily weaken your immune system, leading to gut flora flare ups along with the associated symptoms. (See chapter 8 for more about gut flora and how WBV can help balance these organisms, and chapter 9 for detoxing and how to alleviate detox overdosing.)

3. Hormonal and metabolic imbalances: If you have eliminated the first two causes for not losing weight, you may have hormonal and/or metabolic imbalances. There are numerous hormonal and metabolic issues that can make it difficult to lose weight. Sometimes you can reset your metabolic and hormonal systems with a stringent diet, such as the ketogenic diet or an "intermittent fasting" approach in which you eat only during four to eight hours of the day. Even more drastically, the "Fast-Mimicking Diet," in which you don't eat for several days at a time, has been shown to stimulate stem cells and bring rapid and dramatic health benefits. You can also consult a qualified health professional to address these issues and be sure to check with your doctor before fasting.

Chapter 6

A Healthy Gut = A Calm Immune System

Hippocrates, the father of medicine, believed that all disease began in the gut. Modern science is providing an explanation for what is, indeed, a very close connection. Inflammation, a driving force in nearly all chronic health conditions,[1] is created by the immune system; and the gut is *the* major battleground for immune system activity, with 70–80 percent of immune system activity found in the gut.[2] By focusing on your gut, you can have a powerful impact on inflammatory conditions. For the greatest success with your natural anti-inflammation plan, you should choose at least one (more is better!) gut health method in this book (see chapters 7 and 8) to add to the powerful benefits WBV brings.

Not surprisingly, common signs of gut health issues are digestive system symptoms—leading to digestive distress being among the most common of health issues worldwide, especially in developed countries such as the US. It is estimated that sixty to seventy million Americans, or one out of five people, suffer from chronic digestive diseases[3] in which inflammation is a major factor in the condition. This includes issues such as chronic diarrhea and/or constipation (IBS, IBSD), heartburn and GERD, ulcers, hemorrhoids, diverticulitis, bloating, cramping, ulcerative colitis, Crohn's disease, celiac disease, and others.

The gut is the major battleground for immune system activity, with 70–80 percent of immune system activity found in the gut. By focusing on your gut, you can have a powerful impact on inflammatory conditions.

Inflammation in the gut can eventually cause symptoms all over the body. Overworked and stressed by poor conditions in the gut, the immune system becomes hyperactive and confused and starts creating problems throughout the body. Organs and systems such as the heart and respiratory system can be affected by inflammation originating in the gut. Your immune system may begin attacking benign substances (this is an allergic reaction) and eventually even your own body (autoimmune conditions).

Your immune system is like an army of fighters protecting you, but if soldiers have no sleep or rest for prolonged periods—days, months, or even years on end—they can become triggered too easily. As Amy Myers writes, in her book *The Autoimmune Solution*, "When inflammation becomes chronic, your immune system is like an overworked security squad whose guys have been on the job six straight days without a break. As you can imagine, they are likely to make all sorts of mistakes—with potentially disastrous consequences for your health."[4]

A confused, overworked immune system is why other common early signs of gut inflammation can be as diverse as acne, fatigue, excess weight, and depression. As gut conditions worsen and inflammation levels increase, more serious issues develop, such as asthma, allergies, joint pain, chronic fatigue, and heart disease. At the far end of the inflammation spectrum are autoimmune diseases and possibly even cancers.

WBV was first developed, and is still best known, as an intense workout system, and exercise itself has numerous benefits for the digestive system and gut health. Research has shown that exercise alleviates constipation, improves the absorption of nutrients, lowers stress levels (which lowers inflammation and can thus help numerous digestive and other ills), controls weight (which decreases the risk of gallstones and diabetes), and improves gut flora balance (see chapter 10 for more about the benefits of exercise).

As discussed in the last chapter, WBV also has direct effects on inflammation levels in the gut. There are dramatic increases in beneficial gut flora and immune system cells that suppress inflammation, along with improved levels of key inflammatory cytokines. For the best results, the vibration should be perfectly synchronized, smooth, and calm. This type of vibration is optimal for your nervous system and brain, as well as for your body, helping to lower stress and move your nervous system into a calmer mode where it can focus on digestion and healing.

WBV can also help alleviate constipation and improve digestive system health purely on the mechanical level by increasing peristalsis—the gut lining muscle contractions that move digested materials through your intestines. WBV causes all muscle fibers in the body to automatically tense and relax at the same rate the machine is vibrating—including the muscles that line the digestive tract. Peristalsis is defined by the *Oxford English Dictionary* as "the involuntary constriction and relaxation of the muscles of the intestine that creates wave-like movements that push the contents of the digestive system forward." Perhaps this improvement in peristalsis is why some people report quick improvements for constipation with WBV. Another possibility could be stimulation of the parasympathetic nervous system (which controls digestion and the elimination sphincters) from the relaxation effects of WBV.

Leaky Gut and the Inflammation/Immune System Connection

Consider the task of the gut and your immune system. Every day, billions of particles pass through your digestive system. Your body and immune system must allow only the good particles into your bloodstream, while filtering out and destroying all the dangerous ones. It is a herculean task that our miraculous bodies successfully manage every day—when we are healthy. However, modern life has stacked the deck against our bodies and immune systems with a host of dangerous, damaging conditions, resulting in an epidemic of poor gut health, inflammation, and the chronic health issues that follow.

Normally, the lining of your gut is a tightknit wall of cells that create a strong barricade against unwanted foreign particles moving through your digestive system. If something unhealthy, such as undigested food, bad bacteria, or toxins, does get past this physical barrier and into your bloodstream, your immune system stands at the ready to attack and keep you safe. However, numerous factors in modern life can lead to a weakening of those tight cell wall connections, resulting in a condition called

---

TESTIMONIALS

Two years ago, I decided I had to get serious about my Crohn's disease, as I had been frustrated for years with miserable symptoms despite drugs. I created a program for myself of WBV, meditation, careful eating, and supplements—and I am thrilled to say today that I am off all my drugs and symptom free. Thank you, Becky, for your awesome information and help!

—Michael, age 49

I'm fifty-eight and have Epstein Barr and interstitial cystitis. I use my machine fifteen minutes a day, and it makes me feel great—no matter what my symptoms. It relieves my constipation in fifteen minutes and gives me energy!

Thank you, Becky!

—Lindsey, age 58

"leaky gut," in which unwanted foreign particles leak into your bloodstream. Leaky gut leads to constant war in your gut and for your immune system.[5]

Under normal conditions, with a healthy immune system and gut wall, foreign invaders are relatively rare and quickly dealt with. The battle is short lived, and your body and immune system can relax and calm down between battles. With leaky gut, your immune system is continually leaping into action to defend you against a steady stream of "foreign invaders," creating chronic inflammation.

Numerous factors in modern life can lead to a weakening of those tight cell wall connections, resulting in a condition called "leaky gut," in which unwanted foreign particles leak into your bloodstream. Leaky gut leads to constant war in your gut and for your immune system.

Your small intestine is also where most of your nutrients are absorbed. Twenty feet of small intestines curls compactly in your belly. This section of your digestive system is lined with millions of tiny projections known as villi, which in turn are covered with even smaller hair-like microvilli, giving this twenty-foot section of tubing the square footage of a football field in which to play out its efforts to protect and feed you. A further problem that can occur with leaky gut is damage to the villi and microvilli, leading to less available square footage and thus difficulty absorbing nutrients that are critical for a healthy immune system.

Signs of Leaky Gut

Initially with leaky gut, there may be localized inflammation and discomfort; that is, digestive distress and symptoms. Mental and emotional symptoms are common also. Referred to as the gut-brain connection, these two critical areas are in close communication through the nervous and immune systems, hormones, neurotransmitters, and other molecules produced by gut flora. In fact, up to 90 percent of serotonin, the natural antidepressant, feel-good molecules in your brain, are actually manufactured in the gut.[6] Thus, mental symptoms such as depression, headaches, fogginess, and memory issues can quickly follow gut ills. The connection works the other way around, too; that is, emotional issues can cause gut problems. Because of this close two-way connection, emotional and mental stress will also add fire to inflammation issues.

With continued stress on your body, inflammation worsens, and more problems develop. Food allergies and sensitivities develop as larger undigested food particles start leaking through the gut wall. Normally, the digestive system will break your food down into tiny building-block particles that your immune system understands are good for you. But large food particles look suspiciously like foreign invaders to your immune system, prompting attack. If the gut situation continues to worsen, more serious autoimmune diseases can develop in which the immune system becomes so confused that it begins to attack the body's own tissues.

Causes of Leaky Gut

There are numerous causes of leaky gut, and most are related to modern life. Chief among them are diet and food quality related issues, gut flora imbalances, prescription drugs, toxins, lack of exercise, and stress.[7]

- **Diet and food quality:** Our modern diet of highly processed foods is loaded with unhealthy substances and stripped of the nutrients that our digestive and immune systems need. Practices such as large-scale commercial farming, which rely on GMOs (genetically modified organisms), fertilizers, pesticides, and herbicides, introduce toxins and new forms of food that our gut linings are not designed to deal with and that can cause leaky gut. The best approach is to stay away from highly processed foods; instead, eat whole, unprocessed, ideally organic foods (see chapter 7 for anti-inflammatory diet guidelines).

High quality foods full of nutrients are also critical for healing your immune system and gut lining. Your body uses protein for every new cell it makes—and it is replacing all your cells all the time![iv] You need antioxidants to

---

[iv]About 330 billion cells are replaced daily, equivalent to about 1 percent of all our cells. In eighty to one hundred days, thirty trillion will have been replenished—the equivalent of a new you. (Mark Fischetti and Jen Christiansen, "Our Bodies Replace Billions of Cells Every Day: Blood and the Gut Dominate Cell Turnover," *Scientific American* [April 1, 2021].)

neutralize toxins; healthy fats for hormones, cell walls, and nerve cells; vitamins for catalyzing critical reactions; and many other nutrients. It's a mind-bendingly complex system perfected by mother nature. Our job is just to eat the foods that mother nature provides, in as pure a form as possible, and to take care of our body so it stays healthy and can do its work. If you have already developed inflammation and gut health issues, your body will need extra help to heal. Check out the suggested supplements at the end of chapter 7, and gut flora issues in chapter 8.

- **Gut flora imbalances:** Gut flora refers to the microorganisms (i.e., bacteria and yeasts) that live in your gut. It is hard to believe, but there are actually more bacteria cells in your bodies than human cells—and most of those bacteria live in your gut. Beneficial bacteria in your gut are essential for digestion, metabolism, and even for lowering inflammation. Unfortunately, several modern lifestyle factors, especially in America, have led to an epidemic of imbalance with these organisms—too few good ones and too many bad ones. This imbalance of bacteria and yeast types (and sometimes other parasites) can cause leaky gut and skyrocketing inflammation. It is critical to keep this microflora in a healthy balance. Chapter 8 will explain how to control gut flora with WBV, diet, and supplements.

- **Prescription drugs:** Numerous prescription drugs interfere with proper digestion and gut health, potentially causing leaky gut. These common medications are taken by millions of people daily for symptomatic relief, but they have side effects that can lead to more severe issues over time. The first line of treatment should be the safe and effective natural methods at our fingertips—before entering the trickier zone of drugs. If you are already on drugs, you can often safely reduce or get off drugs by using these natural methods—but this should be done with the help of your doctor.

Drugs that can cause gut flora imbalance and leaky gut[8] include:

Antibiotics, which can kill the good bacteria in your gut along with bad bacteria;

Acid blockers, which decrease the acid in your stomach—but acid is critical for digestion and for protection against bacteria and other intruders[v] (see also chapter 7, Heartburn and Related Conditions, page 91);

Birth control pills, which change the hormonal balance in your body, increasing the level of sugar in your bloodstream, which feeds bad bacteria and yeast.

NSAID anti-inflammatory pain killers (aspirin, ibuprofen, naproxen sodium, and others), which, with long-term use, can damage the mucosal lining of your gut leading to leaky gut,[9] ulcers, and other digestive system disorders;[10]

Prednisone and other steroid drugs, which can suppress the immune system, leaving you vulnerable to gut microorganisms and other dangerous disease organisms; and

Chemotherapy, which has been linked to "increased intestinal wall permeability . . . and the onset of a systemic inflammatory immune response,"[11] according to research

---

[v]The cause of heartburn and a host of related problems is very rarely too much acid in the stomach. The problem stems from the valve between the stomach and the esophagus (the tube through which food travels from your throat to your stomach) not tightening properly and keeping the acid in the stomach, which is designed to handle acid. Your esophagus is not designed to handle acid and therefore it will burn, causing pain and potentially damaging the lining of the esophagus. In the long run, turning off acid production in your stomach will lead to many more health issues as protection from all sorts of parasites, bacteria, viruses, and yeast decreases, and the ability to digest and absorb essential nutrients is crippled. If you have severe or chronic heartburn, consult with a doctor to rule out possible dangerous conditions. The methods in this book can often help heartburn—see also the supplements specifically listed for heartburn at the end of chapter 7 and check out *Natural Alternatives to Nexium, Maalox, Tagament, Prilosec & other Acid Blockers*, by Martie Whittekin, for additional help.

on the long-term effects on gut flora from chemotherapy and other health measures in young adult cancer survivors.

- **Toxins:** Toxins are everywhere. There are over 80,000 chemicals registered for use in the US, including dangerous substances like heavy metals and carcinogens. Some molds that can hide out in our houses or environments can also be a source of serious toxins. Studies by the CDC in the first decade of this century[12] have shown that the average American has over one hundred different toxins in their body. Many toxins are thought to contribute to leaky gut, as well as compromising the immune system in other, more direct ways. (More on toxins in chapter 9.)

- **Lack of exercise:** Modern life has also led to a sedentary lifestyle for many people—but we are designed to move. We need exercise and movement for many functions of our bodies that affect the health of our guts: digestion and metabolism, circulation, stimulation of peristalsis, immune system health and inflammation, gut flora levels, and stress reduction. Exercise is critical for gut health. Whole body vibration is a form of exercise, and that is a godsend for many sedentary people. Ideally, augment your WBV program with other forms of exercise (see chapter 10).

- **Stress:** Stress of any type, including trauma, can contribute to leaky gut. Modern life is loaded with stress—financial stress and the need to work more and harder, health fears, the drive to keep up with the perceived success of others, worries about the climate, wars, the news. Because of the mind/body connection, stress of any sort—from accidents, injuries, surgeries, emotional and sexual traumas, and lower grade but chronic stressors such as a stressful job or personal relationship—can contribute to leaky gut.

This includes childhood trauma and stress, as it is carried with us as we grow and can contribute to illness later in life. Stress reduction methods, including WBV, can help lower inflammation—by helping to heal leaky gut, one of the major causes of inflammation. Additional methods to calm our minds and lower stress will be presented in chapter 11.

The health of our guts is critical for the health of our entire body—and we need to address gut health in order to lower inflammation throughout our bodies.

But first, jump on your vibration machine and get your vibe going! With the improved mood, energy, strength, and lower pain and symptoms that you get from vibration, tackling your diet and other lifestyle factors impacting inflammation will not seem quite so overwhelming.

Chapter 7

A Quick and Easy Anti-Inflammation Food Plan

You are what you eat. If you want a well-functioning body, you need to supply it with pure, whole foods—not overly processed junk food. Since your gut is where chronic inflammation starts, it is not surprising that what you eat can make a world of difference. It can be hard to change what you eat and to stick to your new plan, though; WBV's mood, energy, and hormone boosting effects lessen food cravings, hunger, and emotional overeating.

The same diet that provides the nutrients your body needs to heal will also lower inflammation. Aim for a diet rich in fruits and vegetables, low in carbohydrates, and that has plenty of healthy fats and proteins.

Even if you are eating well, a recovering body and immune system often need extra nutrients. A few well-selected nutritional supplements are recommended to round out your program and make sure you are getting what you need (see the end of this chapter for supplement suggestions). Select your vitamins wisely. Watch out for sugar or other additives, such as with the newly popular vitamin gummies. Added sugar and other sweeteners can increase sugar cravings, sabotaging your efforts.

The guidelines below combine anti-inflammation nutrition with super simple and quick preparation—sometimes none! These are general guidelines for health and lowering gut and body-wide inflammation, applicable to most people. They are especially designed for people who do not have the time, interest, or energy to focus on food and cooking—but still love to eat and need to improve their diet. If you like to cook and are willing to spend more time, there are many wonderful anti-inflammation recipes and cookbooks; check online and in the suggested reading section at the end of this book.

If you have a more serious inflammatory condition, you may require additional programs. Some specific conditions, such as diverticulitis, IBS, Crohn's disease, diabetes, and gut flora issues such as SIBO and *Candida* yeast overgrowth, may have additional or different requirements. Chapter 8 has more information regarding gut flora and food sensitivities. If you have a health condition, please check with your doctor and modify your program as needed.

NOTE: Lowering inflammation by combining these diet guidelines with the programs in chapter 8 can give you the greatest relief, but be aware that constipation issues can worsen initially as part of the healing process. This is because when you have inflammation and irritation in your gut, your body often ends up moving your bowels out of irritation rather than due to a natural rhythm, and eventually you can lose your natural rhythm. Initially, when the irritation/inflammation calms, there could then be little stimulus for bowel movements.

Until your natural rhythm is reestablished, which can take time, you may need additional help. Remember, increasing constipation could be a good sign indicating that you are succeeding in lowering inflammation. But do also check out the end of this chapter for some natural constipation remedies.

Guideline # 1: Fruits and Vegetables

Packed with nutrients and full of flavor, texture, and delight, many fruits and vegetables are delicious just as they are—no cooking required. Try grapes, berries (get organic, since berries can be heavily sprayed with pesticides), apples, peaches, cherry tomatoes, baby carrots, sugar snap peas, bell peppers, green beans . . . there are so many choices. A favorite snack might be a ripe tomato sliced on a gluten- and yeast-free rice cake (this option will also work for a gut flora diet plan—see chapter 8) with a few basil leaves and some goat cheese or just a dab of olive oil. Or a bowl of strawberries and blueberries. Add a handful of raw or roasted nuts, or a piece of cheese, or plain (non-sweetened) yogurt.

If regular cow's milk dairy products are a problem, goat cheese is delicious and may work for you; or, if you prefer a plant-based diet, choose from a wide range of plant-based cheeses, yogurts, and spreads. In this way, you can have a light, healthy, quick and easy anti-inflammatory meal that you can eat at home or on your way to work.

Also stock up on high quality frozen fruits and vegetables (avoid sauces that will have less-healthy ingredients in them). When you have no time, but you still want to eat well, grab a bag of ready-to-go healthy food from the freezer and be ready to eat in minutes.

Avoid foods with added sugar. Plain is good, or you can make your own, more healthily sweetened alternatives—see chapter 8 for healthy sweetener options.

Organic is ideal, but just by eating lower on the food chain (vegetarian food sources), you will be reducing the number of toxins your body has to deal with. You will not only be improving your own inner environment, but you will also be helping the outer environment of our natural world. The extra nutrients will also give your body what it needs to process and neutralize toxins already in your system.

If you want to prepare more elaborate meals, that is great! But don't use time as an excuse—even tired or busy people can still eat well.

Guideline # 2: Whole Foods, Not Processed Foods

Just by eating whole foods (foods as close to their original state as possible)—such as raw fruits and vegetables, nuts and seeds, and small amounts of whole grains and legumes—you will dramatically increase the number of nutrients you are getting.

One orange has fifty important vitamins and nutrients, all working together in a synergistic symphony of health. The type of sugar in fruit (fructose) also will not cause the problems that the sugar in a cookie or candy bar (usually processed cane sugar) will cause. However, any type of sugar can still cause problems for people with some health issues—see chapter 8. Whole fruits and vegetables are perfectly designed by mother nature to build and sustain your life.

Stay away from junk food. Highly processed foods low in nutrients, loaded with unhealthy additives, including added sugars, lead to numerous health problems. For the most part, you should walk right by the entire middle of the supermarket and the bakery. Those areas, full of tempting chips, soda, cookies, cakes, candy, pasta, ice cream, et cetera, are seductive and appealing, but beware, they will sabotage your anti-inflammation plan.

Once you have spent a few weeks eating whole foods, your pallet will begin to savor the taste of real food. (Check chapter 8 for more help in avoiding these foods.) You will not only soon feel better but also your taste buds will rapidly recalibrate so that fruits and vegetables will once again become the sweet, juicy bursts of flavor and texture they are meant to be—nature's gift to you.

TIP: Don't shop when you are hungry or depressed and your willpower is low; your body will naturally crave the most intensive sugars and processed foods. If you do find yourself in the supermarket when you are hungry and tempted, pick up a bag of baby carrots or sugar snap peas and munch on those while you shop to distract yourself and satisfy your craving. If you can keep unhealthy foods out of your home, you will have a much better chance of not eating them. If you live with someone who craves unhealthy food, see if you can get them to help you by keeping these foods out of the home. It could mean a healthier phase for everyone.

And when you shop—stick to the perimeter of the supermarket where the whole foods are—fresh fruits and vegetables, nuts, meat, poultry, fish, and dairy—foods that are full of nutrients, health, and peace for your body.

Guideline # 3: Low Carbohydrates

Low-carb diets are popular right now—with good reason. Too many carbs and sugars, especially in the form of junk foods that contain highly processed grains, can lead to leaky gut, gut flora imbalance, and increased inflammation levels. Many grains, such as wheat, corn, and rye, contain a protein called gluten that can cause leaky gut and lead to food sensitivities and autoimmune conditions such as celiac disease. A small number of whole grain products is usually okay for a healthy person (and gut), but you are playing with fire if you are eating a diet high in processed grains. Sugar feeds the detrimental bacteria and yeast in our guts, leading to overgrowths of these persistent and unwanted invaders.

Low-carb diets will also help you lose and control weight—and as obesity and excess weight contribute to inflammation, a slimmer you will help lower inflammation. Instead of baked goods, pasta, and junk food, get your carbs primarily from fruits and vegetables.

Sugar cravings can be powerful; in fact, sugar can be a true addiction. Sometimes called the "mother of all addictions," sugar effects our brains in a manner similar to alcohol and other addictive substances, triggering the production of serotonin and beta-endorphins—two powerful feel-good molecules that are naturally produced in your brain. Limiting sugar and carbs and balancing carbs with protein can help stabilize serotonin and beta-endorphins—and control sugar cravings.[1] Especially for sugar-sensitive people (maybe most of us?), this can be a godsend.

Too many carbs and sugars can lead to leaky gut, gut flora imbalance, and increased inflammation levels.

If you do not have a gluten or other grain sensitivity, you can have some whole grain products in small quantities—I recommend rice cakes (actually, rice is a grain that is naturally gluten free, so even gluten-sensitive people can have rice—Lundeburg brand are my favorite) and Ryvita rye crackers. These are light, whole-grain crackers that have only a small amount of carbs and no yeast or other ingredients except salt (so also good for gut flora diets—see chapter 8). They make an excellent replacement for bread and pasta. Try spreading these crackers with humas, almond butter, salmon salad, et cetera, and you will have the basis for a quick and delicious meal or snack.

(Check out chapter 8 for additional ways to control sugar cravings and avoid the sugar trap.)

Guideline # 4: Proteins

Protein provides the building blocks for rebuilding your immune system and other tissues in your body. It is a vital nutrient for your body to be able to repair itself and lower inflammation. Be sure to eat some healthy proteins along with your fruits and vegetables. Good sources include animal proteins (poultry, meat, fish, dairy, eggs), nuts and seeds, and beans combined with whole grains. Organic and free-range or grass-fed animals are healthier themselves, which will end up being healthier for you, too. These options are more expensive in the short run but can save you money in the long run—nothing is more expensive than poor health.

Guideline # 5: Healthy Fats

Fats are an important nutrient for health—they are critical for many tissues: cell walls throughout your body are built with fat molecules, and your brain, hormones, nerves, heart, and many other tissues depend on fats. Without healthy fats, our bodies would quickly fall apart, but some fats are much better than others—so choose wisely.

Omega-3 oils have powerful anti-inflammatory properties, along with providing important building blocks for tissues. A review by the American College of Nutrition of numerous clinical trials assessing the benefits of "supplementation with fish oils in several inflammatory and autoimmune diseases in humans, including rheumatoid arthritis, Crohn's disease, ulcerative colitis, psoriasis, lupus erythematosus, multiple sclerosis and migraine headaches . . . reveal significant benefit, including decreased disease activity and a lowered use of anti-inflammatory drugs."[2]

The authors went on to conclude that other health issues, such as coronary heart disease, major depression, aging, and cancer (which are also inflammation-driven conditions), might also benefit from omega-3 supplementation. Unfortunately, other fats, such as omega-6 oils, can increase inflammation, and most people get too much omega-6 and too little omega-3. Following the anti-inflammation diet guidelines for avoiding processed foods will also help you lower omega-6 oils.

Fish and other seafood are a great source of omega-3 oils. However, certain seafoods are also high in toxins, so choose your seafood carefully (see chapter 9 for more on toxins, including which seafood is safer and which ones to avoid). One approach is to limit seafood, and this is especially recommended if you are not careful about what seafood you eat, to no more than once or twice a week and supplement with krill oil (see below). Other good sources of healthy fats are walnuts, flax seeds, and avocados.

Nutritional Supplements

With depleted soils, long transportation times, and other factors leading to lower quality food sources, and especially when nutritional requirements are greater due to healing and repair, taking high quality, targeted supplements can make a big difference. Be careful to read the labels of your supplements to be sure they don't contain items that can trigger reactions in you. In general, follow the dosage guidelines on the container unless otherwise recommended by your doctor.

Please check with a nutritionist or doctor if you are combining different supplements and/or have a health condition. While nutritional supplements are generally very safe and beneficial, it is possible to overdose when combining supplements, especially if you have a health condition. For example, if you combine a vitamin D3 supplement with krill oil, which naturally has vitamin D3 in it, that's a "double dose" of the vitamin. D3 is essential for immune system function, mood, and bones, but too much can lead to kidney stone formation for people predisposed to them.[3]

General Anti-Inflammatory Supplements

These supplements are recommended for everyone interested in reducing inflammation and maintaining and improving their health.

- ♦ **A multi-nutrient protein powder made from whole foods:** A good whole-foods nutritional powder can give you the nutrients of ten or more fruits and vegetables plus protein and a host of other important digestive and immune system nutrients every day—in one shot. If you are up to making your own nutritional drink daily from raw fruits, veggies, herbs, and more, this would be even better, but it is a lot of work, so not always practical for a busy person. Ideally, your nutritional shake should contain *antioxidants* (anti-aging and anti-inflammatory foods), *probiotics and fiber* (for digestive system health), *natural digestive enzymes* (to improve digestion), *super greens* (like algae and wheat grass—full of toxin-fighting and anti-aging chlorophyll, antioxidants, minerals, and vitamins), as well as *protein and omega-3 healthy oils*. A bonanza of nutrients every day.

Amazon sells a good organic plant-based product made from fifty different whole foods called Orgain Organic Protein & Superfoods, which currently sells for around $40 for a two-pound container. NOTE: While there are some carbs in this product that are not on a low FODMAP diet (see appendix 3), you may still improve when taking it, because the benefits to your immune system and gut health can outweigh the slight increase in carbs.

- **Curcumin:** This is a powerful antioxidant for reducing inflammation.

- **Acetyl-Glutathione:** This is a form of glutathione, one of the most powerful antioxidants naturally produced in the body. This combined form is able to remain intact in the gut, greatly improving absorption and activity of orally ingested glutathione.

- **B vitamins, especially B12:** The B vitamins, especially B12, are essential for stress reduction and mental health. The B vitamins are primarily found in animal meats and seafood; B12 is almost exclusively found in these foods—so vegans and vegetarians especially need B12 and a multi-B-vitamin supplement. But vegetarian or not, people under stress don't always eat a well-balanced diet with plenty of B-vitamin foods, so also often need this supplement. Methylated vitamin B supplements are the most easily absorbed form of this essential nutrient. So they are the best, especially for people with inflammatory conditions, as the "methyl" chemical group has also been found to be deficient in inflammatory conditions such as arthritis and IBS.[4] However, please be careful to follow the directions on the package. I would recommend using only low-dose preparations (50mcg of vitamin B12/serving) unless otherwise advised by a doctor, as it is possible to overdo this supplement.

- **Vitamin D3:** Vitamin D is critical for your immune system, mental well-being, and bone health. It is naturally made by our bodies from exposure to the sun, but with poor weather and lavish use of sunscreen, it is common to end up vitamin-D deficient. Vitamin D3 is the natural form of vitamin D that your body makes from sunlight and is thought to be superior at replenishing your body's supply of vitamin D.

- **Magnesium:** Low magnesium intake is linked to chronic inflammation and studies suggest that about 50 percent of Americans are not getting enough daily magnesium.[5] It is involved in more than six hundred reactions in your body, including energy creation, protein formation, gene maintenance, muscle movements, and nervous system regulation.

- **Krill oil:** Krill are tiny ocean crustaceans that are high in an easily absorbed form of anti-inflammatory omega-3 oil. Krill are also low on the food chain, so they are naturally low in toxins. A vegetarian supplemental source for omega-3 oil is flax seeds.

Healing Leaky Gut

- **Seacure** (Pure Formulas brand): These are predigested fish peptides containing L-glutamine and omega-3 oils that are excellent for helping to repair leaky gut.

- **Collagen:** Regular consumption of collagen can help mend and prevent leaky gut. You can use a liquid or powder collagen supplement or foods containing collagen, such as bone broth or gelatin. Ideally use collagen from a grass-fed bovine or goat.

Gut Flora Balancing

It is highly recommended to add the supplements below for balancing gut flora, along with other diet changes (see chapter 8 for specifics on these supplements and other gut flora–balancing methods).

- **Natural yeast- and bacteria-killing products:** Garlic and many other herbs, spices, and foods have anti-yeast and antibacterial properties. Details in chapter 8.
- **Probiotics:** These are the good bacteria that should be in your gut. If you have a problem with gut flora, additional probiotics are highly recommended.
- **GI Microb-X** (Designs for Health brand): *Optional—for other gut parasites.* If you are not having success in calming your gut with the methods in this book, you may have other types of parasites in your gut. Consult with a doctor and consider taking this product, which is a blend of botanical extracts that inhibit several different intestinal parasites.

Natural Remedies for Constipation

- **Xylitol:** This tastes and looks like sugar—but it is not sugar. Xylitol works the way prunes do—so don't use too much! For people who tend toward constipation, Xylitol can be a wonderful product and a healthy alternative to sugar. But be careful, xylitol can cause diarrhea, and some people are very sensitive to it. Try only a small amount at first (less than a teaspoon). Xylitol will not cause cavities in your teeth or problems for diabetics; however, its effects on gut flora are mixed,[vi] and it is a high FODMAP food. FODMAP is a dietary treatment for SIBO (small intestine bacterial overgrowth), which commonly causes IBS (see chapter 8 for more on these subjects).

Corn sourced versions are not advised, as corn is a problematic food choice itself; birch sourced is the best option. Try some in the morning in a cup of coffee or tea for an enjoyable, constipation relieving effect. **Warning:** While xylitol is generally beneficial and safe for humans and most other animals, due to a quirk in their metabolism, **xylitol is extremely toxic for dogs—one teaspoon can rapidly cause death. Be extremely careful to keep xylitol away from dogs.**

- **Crushed flax seeds, or psyllium:** These fibers absorb a lot of water, creating bulk and a slippery mucus, which can make a big difference the next day. Flax seeds are also a good source of omega-3 oils. Take two heaping tablespoons once or twice a day in a large glass of water (drink within a few minutes, or it will not work properly).

- **MgO:** Magnesium oxide is effective for constipation, but be careful; too much can cause diarrhea. Magnesium is an essential element for health and is often deficient, so taking magnesium can also help with numerous other health issues, including muscle and leg cramps, muscle and bone pain, cardiac issues (arrythmias, palpitations, murmurs), high blood pressure, depression, insomnia, and fatigue.

- **Triphala:** This is an Ayurvedic mixture of three herbal medicines that is famous for relieving constipation.

[vi] See the "Safe Sweeteners" section on page 104.

- **Senna:** This is a herbal product that has powerful actions on the large intestine and rectum. Be careful with this herb, as it can easily cause diarrhea.

Heartburn and Related Conditions

Too much stomach acid is rarely the cause of heartburn and related conditions. The goal is not to lower stomach acid—acid is critical for digestion and for protection against bacteria and other intruders. In fact, too *little* stomach acid is often the cause of heartburn because it contributes to undigested food backing up in the digestive system; this causes the sphincter at the top of the stomach, which normally keeps food in the stomach, to not work properly. This allows acidic stomach fluids into the esophagus (the tube that connects the stomach to the mouth). The esophagus is not designed to handle stomach acid and will burn—this is what causes the pain of heartburn, indigestion, GERD, and related issues.

Turning off acid production in your stomach will lead to many more health issues. If you have severe or chronic heartburn, check with your doctor to be sure you do not have a potentially dangerous condition such as a bleeding ulcer. Then, follow the guidelines in this book to address the deeper underlying causes of heartburn, and try the products below to soothe and protect your GI tract while you are addressing the root of the problem. Also check out *Natural Alternatives to Nexium, Maalox, Tagament, Prilosec and Other Acid Blockers*, by Martie Whittekin, for further natural methods to alleviate stomach acid–related health issues.

- **DGL (Deglycyrrhizinated Licorice):** Licorice is an herbal supplement that can be extremely useful in healing stomach issues. DGL is a form of licorice that is very safe. DGL has had the glycyrrhizin component removed, as glycyrrhizin can cause high blood pressure and water retention. DGL strengthens and helps to heal the lining of the GI tract. In fact, it can have nearly the same success rate in healing ulcers as acid blocking drugs do.[6] I find the chewable DGL tablets made by Planetary Herbals particularly effective for occasional discomfort, though they do not use ideal sweeteners. For chronic issues, you can take a different brand of unsweetened DGL capsules daily before meals.

- **Zinc-Carnosine:** These two products synergistically adhere to damaged areas in the intestinal tract and form a protective barrier against stomach acid without reducing stomach acid—which you do not want to do.

- **Calcium:** Calcium can help strengthen the action of the sphincter that is meant to keep stomach acid out of your throat. Counterproductively, acid blockers inhibit the absorption of calcium. For heartburn, as well as for strong bones, try taking a good balanced source of minerals. I recommend Pure Synergy Bone Renewal, which is a low-toxicity, natural, algae-based mineral supplement that contains a range of important minerals for many bodily functions, as well as for bone health.

Chapter 8

Balancing Gut Flora

It is hard to believe, but there are more bacteria and other micro flora in our bodies than there are human cells—and most of those microorganisms live in our guts. The result is that 70–80 percent of your immune system is actually in your GI tract. If you want to lower inflammation, creating a healthy balance of gut flora is an excellent place to start—and WBV can help you.

Gut flora balance can easily be upset by modern lifestyle practices, with disastrous effects on your body over time, but you can fix this situation. **By changing your diet and lifestyle, you can kill off large amounts of bad gut flora.** These bad players are also a major cause of leaky gut, so you will be helping your gut to heal from other inflammation producing conditions as well.

Try the following program to improve your gut health and receive a host of benefits—including improved mental health and weight loss. And don't forget to also use your WBV machine! WBV can be a powerful ally in balancing gut flora. WBV has been shown to potentially lead to a seventeen-fold increase in the numbers of critical bacteria in the gut that calm inflammation and increase immune system cells that, in turn, produce anti-inflammatory effects (see chapter 3). WBV also lowers stress, which will help your immune system to fight this battle more effectively.

> *WBV can be a powerful ally in balancing gut flora. WBV has been shown to potentially lead to a seventeen-fold increase in the numbers of critical bacteria in the gut that . . . produce anti-inflammatory effects.*

SIBO and *Candida* Yeast Overgrowth

Poor diets with few nutrients and too much sugar, the overuse of certain drugs,[vii] too little exercise, toxins, and high stress levels can play havoc with the balance of gut flora. These factors lead to weakened immune systems and the perfect conditions in your gut for unhealthy microorganisms to flourish. SIBO, a bacterial overgrowth in the small intestine, and fungal (*Candida* yeast) overgrowths in the small and large intestines are the most common culprits.

SIBO and yeast overgrowths are at epidemic levels in modern life. Common symptoms from these conditions include

---

[vii] As mentioned earlier, numerous drugs can affect gut health and gut flora balance. Drugs to particularly avoid include antibiotics, acid blockers, birth control pills, NSAIDs, and steroids such as prednisone (see page 74 for details).

depression and anxiety, digestive system problems, bloating and water retention, allergies, fatigue, and a long list of other issues.[1]

Some of the gut and body symptoms are the result of the inflammation that comes as your immune system attacks these unwanted residents, a type of inflammation reaction that commonly causes diarrhea, pain, and cramping. Symptoms can also result from toxic effects of fermentation as these bacteria and yeasts consume sugars in your gut. Consider the fermentation process when making bread or beer—there is a lot of gas and alcohol produced in these processes. Another cause of IBS symptoms can be the osmotic water-attracting effects of some foods (e.g., prunes).

Take the SIBO and Candida *yeast quiz at the end of this chapter to see if these gut flora imbalances are likely to be a problem for you.*

Bacterial and yeast overgrowths have many symptoms and risk factors in common; the result is that if you have one, there is a good chance you may have the other as well. As the treatment is similar for both conditions, it can be wise to address both at once.[2]

Take the SIBO and *Candida* yeast quiz at the end of this chapter to see if these gut flora imbalances are likely to be a problem for you. As these gut flora imbalances are so prevalent in the US, taking preventative countermeasures is always a good idea—especially for people with inflammation issues. You can get tests from a doctor to determine if you have one or both of these conditions, but testing is not particularly reliable for *Candida* due to various reasons.[viii] One of the most effective ways to determine if you have a gut flora issue is to try the steps below for a few weeks, then see if you feel better. You can also confirm your results, after your gut has calmed down, by reintroducing foods one at a time and seeing how you react to them.

Three Steps to Balance Your Gut Flora Naturally

Bad bacteria and yeast are like weeds in a garden—they always grow unless the garden (your gut) is full of desirable plants (the good bacteria), and there is a healthy gardener (your immune system) to pull up the weeds (the bad bacteria and yeast). A small amount of *Candida* yeast is actually a normal inhabitant of a healthy colon, but it can easily overgrow and cause trouble. For most people, and for long-term health, the best way reestablish healthy gut flora is with a gentle natural approach with three goals:

1. kill the bad gut flora,

2. repopulate your gut with probiotics, and

3. starve the bad gut flora by cutting back sugar.

[viii] A simple antibody blood test for *Candida* is not very reliable. A "*Candida* immune complex" test, which looks for *Candida* bound to antibodies, is more accurate. However, while Western medicine is currently enthusiastic about diagnosing SIBO as a cause of digestive ills, conventional Western medicine is still reluctant to recognize *Candida* yeast as a major player in chronic gut health issues. Thus, your doctor may not think that *Candida* yeast could be contributing to your health issues. On the other hand, natural health doctors have recognized *Candida* yeast as a significant cause of gut and other symptoms for many years.

Whole body vibration (WBV) can be critical for success, especially long term, because WBV strengthens your immune system along with the rest of your body, and a strong immune system is essential for establishing and maintaining a healthy gut flora balance. Powerful antifungal and antibiotic prescription drugs should be avoided unless absolutely necessary because, long term, their higher toxicity level can weaken the immune system; a strong immune system is one of the three critical conditions for long-term healthy gut flora balance.

As part of your program, try to eat more mindfully and slowly. Enjoy your food. Don't gulp; instead, chew and savor. And try not to overstuff yourself. These things can improve your digestive system functions. Luckily, sugar and food cravings should decrease as your mood and health improves with WBV, a better diet, and balanced gut flora, making this mindful and more enjoyable approach to eating more natural and easier. As emotional stress can also set off IBS, the mood-enhancing effects of WBV can be valuable here as well.

The following three-pronged natural program, plus WBV, addresses the three goals above. Everyone should add steps 1

> *Whole body vibration can be critical for success because WBV strengthens your immune system along with the rest of your body, and a strong immune system is essential for establishing and maintaining a healthy gut flora balance.*

and 2 below to their anti-inflammation health plan—they are so easy; add two natural supplements to your daily routine: garlic (or another natural antibiotic/antifungal product) and probiotics (the good bacteria that should be in your gut). Changing your diet by reducing sugar (step 3) is harder, but it can yield big results.

> *Everyone should add steps 1 and 2 to their anti-inflammation health plan—they are so easy; add two natural supplements to your daily routine: garlic and probiotics.*

Go Slow: I recommend implementing your gut flora plan slowly, over the course of a few weeks. This is because killing off large amounts of these microorganism can cause a "die-off" reaction that may initially cause you to you feel worse. This happens because as the yeast or bad bacteria cells die, they break apart and release stored toxins into your body. If this happens too quickly, you can feel a lot worse before feeling better. *Try step one the first week, add step two the second week, then step three the third week.*

Gut Flora Balancing Plan Steps

1. **Kill the bad gut flora:** There are many safe natural products that have antibacterial and antifungal properties. You can try any of the following products or a combination of them. These and others are available in natural health stores and online.

   Allicin: An extract of garlic that is both antibacterial and antifungal. While whole garlic contain the sugars that can feed bad bacteria, allicin does not. Garlic is not allowed on the FODMAP diet (which is often recommended for SIBO and IBS—see below), but allicin is fine. Brand names include Kyolic and Allimed.

Berberine complex: Contains berberine, an antibacterial compound found in Oregon grape, barberry, goldenseal, and other herbs

Caprylic acid: An antibacterial and antifungal coconut extract

Grapefruit seed extract: Antibacterial and antifungal (not to be confused with grapeseed extract)

Oregano leaf extract: Antibacterial and antifungal

Pau d'arco: An antibacterial and antifungal tea made from bark of the pau d'arco tree.

2. **Repopulate your gut with probiotics:** Probiotics are the good bacteria that should be in your gut. Be sure to add a generous daily source of these to your program. There are many probiotic supplements available (see below for recommended products). Look for one that includes five or more bacterial strains and at least ten billion viable bacteria per serving. Fermented foods are also a good option.

    Physicians Choice 60 Billion Probiotic: Good for both men and women. Currently available on Amazon for $22 for a one-month supply.

    Surebounty 4-in-1 Feminine Probiotic: Numerous bacteria strains equaling 120 billion bacteria per serving, plus digestive enzymes and other nutrients that help with the gut and female health. Currently available on Amazon for $19 for a one-month supply.

    BioK yogurt: This product is good for difficult cases. It is an extra potent (but also expensive) source of live probiotics.

Bacterial fermented foods (good for milder cases):[ix] Check the ingredients lists—products with little to no sugar are best. Examples of these foods include: Activia yogurt, specially prepared raw sauerkraut and kimchi (fermented vegetable products), and kefir and kombucha drinks.

Yeast fermented foods (can be a big problem for some people): These are foods that are fermented with yeast, such as breads, vinegars,[x] alcohol, and soy sauce. Foods made with these items, such as mayo, will also contain yeast. If you have a yeast overgrowth in your gut, avoiding these foods (along with other foods in the fungal family) can yield big results—but fully eliminating these foods is difficult and may not be necessary. First try reducing sugars (see step 3), and if you are still not feeling better after a week, try avoiding bread and alcohol. If you feel better after a week of no bread and alcohol[xi] and want to try a stricter anti-yeast approach, see appendix 4.

3. **Starve the bad gut flora by cutting back sugar:** Bacteria and yeast feed on sugar, so by controlling sugar, you can

---

[ix]These foods often also contain other microorganisms, fibers, and sugars that can cause problems if you already have gut health issues. Some people will do better to start with supplements, then switch to these foods after they have healed their gut.

[x]Apple cider vinegar is often promoted as good for gut flora issues and digestive system health. The idea is that it will increase stomach acid, which will help kill bad bacteria. But I do not recommend any vinegar for gut flora issues, including apple cider vinegar. Using vinegar is not a very effective method for reestablishing gut flora health (Nilgün H. Budak, Elif Aykin, Atif C. Seydim, et al., "Functional Properties of Vinegar," *Journal of Food Science* 79, no. 5 (May 2014): R757–64, https://doi.org/10.1111/1750-3841.12434; Doug Cook, "Apple Cider Vinegar for Digestion. What's the Deal?" Canadian Digestive Health Foundation, https://cdhf.ca/health-lifestyle/apple-cider-vinegar-for-digestion-whats-the-deal.), and all vinegar contains yeast, so if you have a yeast issue wherein your immune system is primed to attack any yeast, apple cider vinegar is likely to also trigger problems. **Fresh lemon juice is an excellent and safe replacement for vinegar.**

[xi]Some people may end up experiencing a lot of ups and downs after eliminating bread and alcohol. Since you are not fully eliminating all other sources of yeast, your immune system could react strongly to those other sources. If at least some of the time you feel better, a stricter program may help you.

starve them out of your body. This is a surprisingly effective approach. In fact, if you have a significant gut flora issue and do not cut back on sugar, you may not see much change. Cutting back on sugar is hard but worth the effort. Below are some options that can help you reduce the sugar that gut flora feeds on, including some safe natural sugar substitutes that will not cause gut flora problems—see the "Safe Sweeteners" section below.

NOTE: If limiting sugar seems impossible, don't despair; after just a week or two of not eating sugar and controlling the gut microflora, sugar cravings should rapidly decrease. And, if you are seriously addicted to sugar and giving it up seems impossible, it probably means this step is extra important for you.

> ***Bacteria and yeast feed on sugar, so by controlling sugar, you can starve them out of your body. This is a surprisingly effective approach.***

FODMAP DIET

FODMAP stands for "fermentable oligosaccharides, disaccharides, monosaccharides, and polyols," meaning fermentable sugars—those sugars that are not easily digested by people and thus end up in the gut longer and fermented by gut microorganisms. This diet is often recommended for SIBO (and resulting IBS) and separates foods based on the type of sugars they contain. Most digestion and absorption of nutrients happens in the small intestine, but because these sugars are not easily absorbed, they can end up in the large intestine.[xii] The sugars can cause water to be drawn into the large intestine through osmosis (similar to the effect of prunes), and they can be rapidly fermented by microorganisms, producing gas. The result may be irritation, inflammation, pain, gas, cramping, diarrhea, and constipation; that is, IBS.

The idea of the FODMAP diet is to selectively reduce these more problematic sugars. For example, on this diet you should not eat *high* FODMAP fruits, such as apples, cherries, pears, and peaches. *Low* FODMAP fruits, including grapes, oranges, strawberries, blueberries, and pineapple, are allowed more freely. See appendix 3 for more low and high FODMAP foods. There are also many online resources and books for more extensive information about the FODMAP diets and how best to follow them. See also the reference section at the end of this book.

However, people differ, and the research on FODMAP is ongoing. Some foods will be okay in small amounts but not larger amounts. There is an element of individual tolerance. The diet works by eliminating foods. It is strict at first, then you gradually reintroduce foods to see which ones you can and cannot tolerate.[xiii]

There is also a handy cellphone app that has extensive lists of FODMAP-categorized foods available at the touch of a finger

---

[xii]There are different types of sugar, and carbohydrates are actually chains of linked sugars that your body separates into single, or simple, sugars during digestion. Most human digestion and absorption happens in the mouth, stomach, and small intestine before food reaches the large intestine

[xiii]Exactly which sugars and carbohydrates cause you problems may depend on what populations of bacteria you have in your gut. Some bacteria preferentially ferment particular types of sugars. Individual tolerance can also stem from the severity of the gut flora imbalance and resulting immune system reactivity.

(Monash University FODMAP diet app: https://www.monash fodmap.com/ibs-central/i-have-ibs/get-the-app).

Candida yeast issues also commonly cause IBS and other issues.[xiv] To control *Candida* yeast, a FODMAP plan can help you transition to a healthier diet and lower overall sugar consumption. However, as almost all sugars will feed yeast, a more comprehensive approach may be needed for yeast-related issues, especially for more severe situations (see appendix 4). *Certain symptoms are highly indicative of yeast issues—see the quiz at the end of this chapter for tips on which ones to watch for.*

Go Light on Carbohydrates

Carbohydrates are broken down in your digestive system into sugars, so they also can feed microorganisms.[xv] For example, do not eat spaghetti, as it is a very carbohydrate-dense food. Instead, have a couple of the Lundberg rice cakes or Ryvita rye crackers that I mentioned in chapter 7 (both of these crackers are also made without yeast, which is good for people with a yeast overgrowth) with some hummus, cheese, or almond butter on them. If you can't eat grains because of food sensitivities, try winter squashes or a small potato. For under ten dollars, you can get a cutting device that makes a delicious spaghetti out of squash, or

---

[xiv]*Candida* yeast is still controversial in Western medicine, but some natural health–oriented doctors believe that *Candida* yeast in the large intestine is the primary cause of IBS.

[xv]Too many carbohydrates at one time can be a problem for yeast issues, as they are then turned into large amounts of sugar during digestion. However, smaller amounts of carbs are less problematic for yeast than simple sugars (such as those in fruit, cane sugar, and other sweeteners) because breaking carbohydrates down into simple sugars during digestion takes time, which allows your immune system to control the situation. Larger amount of carbohydrates can cause problems for both bacteria and yeast.

just buy "spaghetti squash," a type of squash that, after cooking, comes out of the gourd in long spaghetti-like strands.

SAFE SWEETENERS

There are some natural sweeteners that are okay for many but not all people. Two of my favorites are below. Do not use artificial sweeteners; they can have bad long-term effects. You can try using the sweeteners below to make your own flavored yogurt or other treats and see how you do with them. Try adding one heaping teaspoon of the diluted stevia mixture I describe below to one quart of plain yogurt, then flavor with half a teaspoon of vanilla extract or one to two teaspoons of fresh-squeezed lemon juice.

- **Stevia:** Stevia has no calories and is one hundred times sweeter than sugar. It will not raise blood sugar levels—but use it very sparingly, as it has a bitter aftertaste. Pure stevia extract is too concentrated to deal with easily, so I cut pure stevia with goat milk lactose. Mix one part pure powdered stevia (available online or at Whole Foods) with approximately ten times that amount of powdered goat lactose (from www.MtCapra.com). If you can't tolerate lactose (some people can have gut flora problems from this type of sugar), you can use undiluted stevia, but be very sparing—try just a pinch instead of a teaspoon.

- **Monk fruit extract:** This is a calorie- and carbohydrate-free natural sweetener made from monk fruit, native to Southeast Asia. Monk fruit also contains antioxidant compounds that can help support your health and anti-inflammation plan. Do be careful, though, to check the ingredient label, as many monk fruit extract products are combined with sugar or other sweeteners, which you are trying to avoid.

- **Xylitol:** This tastes and looks like cane sugar, but it is not cane sugar and can be a healthy alternative for some people. There are, however, mixed results with Xylitol, and it is a high FODMAP food. Some research shows that it can lower levels of some bad bacteria in the gut[3] as well as in the mouth;[4] other research shows that it can feed bad bacteria. As it is a high FODMAP food, you may find that it does not work for you.[5] But as there is variability for people with FODMAP foods, and it often does not cause yeast to grow, the best approach may be to try a small amount and see how you do with it. Xylitol can be especially helpful for people with yeast overgrowths and constipation, as it works the way prunes do but does not feed yeast the way prunes do. **Do not use Xylitol if you have issues with diarrhea—and try less than a teaspoon the first time to see how you react.**

    NOTE: *Xylitol is extremely toxic for dogs—keep away from dogs.*

The hardest part of a gut flora plan is changing your diet. But if gut flora imbalance is a significant part of your chronic inflammation, the rewards can be rapid and dramatic and often include weight loss, reduced pain, and an improved mood—all of which are highly motivating. Give this food program a try for a few weeks and see what happens.

Using WBV regularly can help you in your effort to eliminate sugar. Many people use sugar as an antidepressant because it gives them a temporary boost or high. But this high is followed by a crash, so it is a disappointing and self-defeating antidepressant in the long run. WBV gives you a lift with no crash afterward—unless you overdo it, so go slow.

Remember, because WBV is such a powerful healing force, you will likely not need to be as strict with the diet or have to follow it for as long. The idea is to give your immune system and gut lining a chance to heal and recover by creating conditions in your gut that the bad flora cannot easily survive. Giving yourself lots of nutrients and health-promoting stimulation with WBV will help this. A healthy immune and digestive system should be fully capable of keeping gut flora in balance. Once you have healed your gut and immune system, you will be able to eat a normal healthy diet, such as the anti-inflammatory plan in chapter 7.

Understanding Your Gut Flora Program Results

If you see significant positive changes, especially if breaking the diet guidelines leads to a quick return of symptoms, it is likely that SIBO and/or yeast is an issue for you.

If, on the other hand, you do not see any changes after a few weeks of adhering to this program, most likely gut flora imbalance is not a major issue for you. If you saw some improvement, but it is a rocky road and you are still having problems, it is possible that you need a stricter gut flora diet plan to give you relief—see appendix 4.

You may also have developed food sensitivities that are causing trouble, as can commonly happen with leaky gut. There are online tests available to check for sensitivities to foods containing gluten, dairy, corn, cane sugar, and many other ingredients.

You can also consult with a natural-health doctor for help with this and other possible gut-health issues.

Hyper-reactivity and Sticking to the Diet

Clearing your body of bad gut flora can bring peace to your immune system and thus to your gut and body. But while you are healing (which can take months or possibly longer), if you break the program, your immune system will still be primed and loaded to attack the bad guys. If you go off your diet, you may suddenly (almost immediately or up to twenty-four hours later) have a major immune-system reaction and feel worse. This can be a blessing in disguise. Hyper-reactivity is great for helping you stick to the diet and letting you know what you need to avoid. You will basically be carrying a carrot and stick with you wherever you go; you will feel great—and possibly lose weight—as long as you follow your diet, but quickly ill when you break it. It is also helpful when you can eat a previously problematic food with no reaction—then you will know you are healing.

Remember, because WBV is such a powerful healing force, you will likely not need to be as strict with the diet or have to follow it for as long.

Quick Relief from Uncomfortable Gut Flora Reactions

If you do have an uncomfortable gut flora reaction, these two measures can help alleviate it.

1. **An extra dose of your probiotics and antifungal, antibacterial products** (those listed in steps 1 and 2 of the gut flora plan). If taking an extra dose of those products gives you relief, this is an additional clue that bad gut flora is contributing to your problems.

2. **Alka-Seltzer Gold.** This product contains only safe, natural bicarbonates and citric acid that will neutralize the pH, or acid/base balance, of your digestive system. (Do not use Alka-Seltzer Blue, as it also contains aspirin, and you should avoid drugs when possible.) Alka-Seltzer Gold (available on Amazon) can relieve many sorts of gut-related immune-system reactions, but it will last only for a few hours, so this is a temporary fix and not a good plan for long-term relief. For long-term relief, you need to follow the three steps of the gut flora plan. But, for emergencies, take two tablets of Alka-Selzer Gold in a large glass of water (drink when dissolved but still fizzy for the best effect).

SIBO and *Candida* Yeast Quiz

Below is a simple SIBO and *Candida* evaluation questionnaire that I have adapted and combined from questionnaires in Amy Myers's *The Autoimmune Solution*[6] and Ann Boroch's *The Candida Cure*.[7] More sophisticated versions are available online and in other literature on the subject. In this questionnaire, give yourself one point for each symptom you currently have or have had in the past and one point for each yes answer. If your score is over 4, there is a good chance you have some issues with gut flora and that this program is likely to help you. If your score is above 8, the changes that come with balancing gut flora could be dramatic, and you might also want to check out the information in appendix 4 for more severe gut flora situations.

Symptom that are particularly indicative of a *Candida* yeast overgrowth are noted at the end of the quiz.

Health History

- Have you taken a lot of antibiotics? This means more than one continuous month of antibiotics or more than four shorter courses of antibiotics in one year.
- Have you taken birth control pills for more than one year or been pregnant several times?
- Have you taken cortisone type drugs by mouth or inhalation?
- Do you crave sugar (cookies, cakes, donuts, pastries, candy, chocolate, ice cream . . . any products with added sugars)? Breads, pasta, pizza? Alcohol?
- Are your symptoms worse on damp, muggy days or in moldy places?
- Have you taken prescription acid blockers or NSAID pain killers for long periods of time; i.e., more than one month?
- Have you been diagnosed with an autoimmune disease, such as Hashimoto's thyroiditis, rheumatoid arthritis, ulcerative colitis, lupus, psoriasis, scleroderma, or multiple sclerosis?

Symptoms

Give yourself a point for every symptom listed below, not just one for each category.

- **Neurological:** sugar, carbohydrate, and alcohol cravings; irritability, mood swings; headaches, migraines; "foggy" feeling, inability to concentrate, poor memory, confusion, dizziness; slurred speech; loss of muscle coordination; affected vision; depression and/or anxiety, mental incompetence, other behavioral disturbances

- **Allergies:** foods and/or airborne chemicals, pollens, molds—especially if these are acquired in adulthood
- **Fatigue and pain:** chronic fatigue, often more noticeable after eating; fibromyalgia; achy joints
- **Gastrointestinal:** poor digestion, constipation or diarrhea, gas (especially gas that smells particularly bad), bloating, cramps, heartburn, nausea, gastritis, colitis
- **Genito-urinary:** vaginal infections, menstrual difficulties, impotence, infertility, prostatitis, rectal itch, urinary tract infection or inflammation, symptoms of urgency or burning, rectal or vaginal itching
- **Respiratory:** lowered resistance (easily catches the flu, colds), hay fever, mucous congestion, postnasal drip, asthma, bronchitis, chest pain, frequent clearing of the throat, habitual coughing (usually nonproductive), sore throat, earaches
- **Skin:** persistent athlete's foot, jock itch, skin rash, eczema, hives, dry brownish patches, rosacea, psoriasis, ringworm, rough skin on sides of arms
- **Clinical history (early childhood):** hyperactivity, aggressiveness, cradle cap, diaper rash, thrush, chronic ear infection, tonsillitis, colic
- **Other symptoms:** feeling bad all over, cold extremities, arthritis-like symptoms, white coating on tongue upon waking, alcoholism

Symptoms Particularly Indicative of a *Candida* Yeast Overgrowth

Candida yeast is an opportunistic parasite, meaning that it takes advantage of a weakened immune system to become established in your body. A healthy body and immune system should be able to fight off yeast and other fungal infections anywhere in or on the body. If you have any persistent fungal infections on the outside of your body, or on mucosal surfaces inside the body such as in your mouth or genital areas, it is likely you have had a *Candida* yeast overgrowth in your gut for years that has weakened your immune system's ability to fight fungal infections everywhere. Follow the guidelines in this chapter and check out appendix 4 and/or one of the *Candida* yeast books in the Suggested Reading section.

- **Fungal infections inside or on the outside of the body:** athlete's foot, ringworm, toenail fungus, vaginal yeast infections, jock itch, oral thrush, rectal itching, yeast or fungal skin rashes
- Gastrointestinal gas that smells particularly bad
- Symptoms worsen after eating yeast-containing foods such as alcohol, vinegar, and breads

My Gut Flora Story

I had to stay on a strict *Candida* yeast diet for about thirty years. During that time, with the exception of a few periods when I was on an upswing, if I broke the diet, I would have painful symptoms within a few hours. I do not believe I would have ever been able to get off this severely restricted diet if not for WBV.

For the last ten years, I have mostly been able to eat normally without getting ill. But because I had such a severe situation for so long, I continue with my gut flora supplements and a gut flora maintenance program in which I eat an anti-inflammatory, whole-foods diet (no junk food) and avoid foods containing yeast and mold.

Most of the time, I feel well and can eat as much fruit and other healthy sugars as I like, and I can occasionally break the diet for special events without a problem. *Candida* yeast issues do still resurface every once in a while, but they are minor, and I can quickly get the situation under control.

Gut flora issues can come and go with stress and poor lifestyle conditions. Like weeds in a garden, they come back. But now you have the knowledge and power to change the situation. Listen to your body—it seeks health and happiness for you.

Chapter 9

Detoxing with Whole Body Vibration

Our environment is loaded with toxins, and despite our best attempts to avoid them, some of these toxins will end up in our bodies. Once in our body, toxins can cause damage and disease, including inflammation. By reducing the "toxic load" in our bodies, we can reduce inflammation, and other damage from toxins, alleviating symptoms and disease. Whole body vibration is a powerful detoxification system, along with its many other benefits. As such, it is a valuable addition to any detoxification program.

Toxins are everywhere. In a PBS television special twenty years ago,

> *By reducing the "toxic load" in our bodies we can reduce inflammation, alleviating symptoms and disease. Whole body vibration is a powerful detoxification system.*

Bill Moyers, as a typical healthy person, had his blood tested at Mt. Sinai School of Medicine. Eighty-four different and highly toxic chemicals were found in his body.[1] A few years later, a study with 2,500 participants by the Centers for Disease Control and Prevention (CDC) confirmed these disturbing results, finding evidence of over 116 chemicals in the participants' bodies.[2] Particularly damaging, and also easily encountered in our environments, are heavy metals, a type of toxin with infamously detrimental effects on the nervous and immune systems.

What to Do

A regular detoxification program is a wise idea for everybody and essential for people with chronic inflammation. Detoxification should be done with caution, though. Detoxing is stressful for the body, and stress itself can cause inflammation, especially in an already weakened body. Your body has natural systems—colon, liver, kidneys, lymphatic system, lungs, and skin—to eliminate and neutralize toxins. Natural methods can assist and support the body in removing toxins through these systems, but with the buildup of toxicity levels in your body and the consequent breakdown of health, it is important to go slowly with detoxing and support your detoxification organs and systems with nutrition and other supplements.

> *A regular detoxification program is a wise idea for everybody and essential for people with chronic inflammation.*

Along with WBV, watching what you eat is at the top of the list of things to do. Our modern diet of highly processed foods is loaded with unhealthy substances and has been stripped of the nutrients that our bodies and immune systems need to mitigate the damage toxins cause. Practices such as large-scale commercial farming—which rely on GMOs (genetically modified organisms), fertilizers, pesticides, and herbicides—degrade the quality of our food. Highly processed food, or "junk food," contains elevated amounts of unhealthy sugars, salt, and fats, along with toxic substances. The best approach is to stay away from highly processed foods. Instead, eat whole, unprocessed foods grown as naturally as possible (organic is best).

Another important guideline is to try to eat low on the food chain. Toxin levels increase rapidly as you move up the food chain, so eating fewer animal products will protect you, and if you are eating animal products, it is even more important to eat from organic and natural sources.

Particularly high in toxins, including heavy metals (see page 121 for more on these dangerous toxins), are fish that are high on the food chain (tuna, swordfish, maki), shellfish and other bottom dwellers, and dark-meat fish such as sardines, bluefish, and herring. Also be aware that most farmed fish is loaded with antibiotics and not as healthy as wild-caught fish. I love seafood, and it is tough to accept that it is not always safe to eat anymore, but I have seen that this is true and that it pays to be careful with what was once a perfect food source.

Happily, some grocery stores, such as Whole Foods, are making great efforts to farm seafood in a sustainable and healthy manner. Whole Foods supplies salmon and shrimp, for example, that are farmed without antibiotics, added growth hormones, or synthetic parasiticides and have been fed no poultry or mammalian products. Salmon and shrimp farmed under these conditions should be relatively safe and low in toxins.

Whole Body Vibration for Detoxing

A key benefit of vibration is that it is a powerful aid to your natural detoxification process. The lymphatic system is a network of vessels, nodes, and organs that removes waste products and toxins from your body, and it is part of your immune-system functions that protect you against infection and disease. This system relies on passive circulation. In other words, unlike the blood vessels (which require a heart to pump the blood through them), there is no pump for the lymphatic system. The lymphatic system relies on your muscles tightening and relaxing around the lymph vessels to move the lymph (a clear fluid), a process called lymph drainage. To keep this system working well, it is important that you use your muscles regularly—something WBV does for you automatically. Even just standing on a vibrating plate will tighten and relax muscles, causing lymphatic drainage.

Even just standing on a vibrating plate will tighten and relax muscles, causing lymphatic drainage.

Many people think they should use powerful, high-amplitude vibration to get as much lymphatic drainage and movement as possible. *Do not do that.* **Slow and steady is the best approach. Too much detoxing too quickly can make you feel worse.** This problem is more common than many realize, especially when using vibration machines with people who already have health problems.

Liberating toxins from where they are relatively safely stored in your body causes a sudden increase in work for your detox organs (liver and kidneys primarily), putting a strain on already overworked and stressed organs. This can lead to increased symptoms instead of relief. I have seen excessive detoxing innumerable times, including in myself.

You do not need high-amplitude vibration for lymphatic drainage and detoxing—any vibration that travels throughout your entire body will be effective for this. In twenty years of using vibration, I have *never* had a person *not* get enough detoxification, including clients with lymphedema (a sometimes painful swelling of arms or legs as lymph builds up in the tissues) and lipedema (an accumulation of excess fat in the legs)—two conditions for which improving lymphatic drainage is particularly important.

The position you hold on the plate determines which muscles are activated, so I advise using a variety of positions. See chapter 13 for photos of different exercise positions. Standing straight up on the Power 1000 machine that I developed will send a strong vibration through your whole body—up through your hips, abdomen and internal organs, your back, and into your head. In fact, you will feel your eyeballs vibrating—enough so that you will not be able to read while standing on this machine.

To increases lymphatic drainage in your arms, you need to get your hands or arms on the plate. You can do some exercise positions in which your hands are on the plate, such as push-ups, or you could rest your arms on the plate for a massage, which will also increase the lymphatic drainage there, as the muscles will still be automatically tensing and relaxing.

WBV Detox Overload

Detoxing with WBV is so powerful that it is the major limiting factor for most people using WBV, not muscle strength as many people assume. Detoxing will happen anytime you are on a machine, whether you just stand there or are actively exercising. As with detoxing after a massage or sauna or any other detox system, it is possible to overload your already stressed detox pathways and have a temporary increase in symptoms. Common detox symptoms are exhaustion, headaches, and digestive problems, but any health issue that is linked to toxins can temporarily worsen as more toxins are released into the circulatory system.

In fact, as any health problem you already have is a "weak link" in your system, when you overstress your body with detoxing, that weak link is a likely place to show the strain. This can result in a sudden and unnerving worsening of the very problem you were worried about and hoping to improve. If this happens, as long as the issue is not a WBV contraindication (see appendix 5 for a list of contraindications), you are probably just doing too much vibration. Stop vibrating and see below for troubleshooting. Detox reactions are an enlightening opportunity to see the close connection between toxins and chronic health issues.

Detox Troubleshooting

Detox problems often do not show up until six to twenty-four hours after using WBV. So even though the vibration feels like a pleasant massage, use caution! Start slowly and increase slowly; many people will do best by starting with just one minute on a gentle, relatively low-power machine (see chapters 12 and 13 for machines and guidelines on getting started).

If any existing symptoms worsen, or new ones suddenly appear, it is possible that toxins are involved. If this happens, you should stop vibrating and rest for a few days; if the symptoms decrease, you can start up again using less vibration. You can aid your body with detoxing by drinking extra water to help flush out toxins and by getting plenty of sleep. Additionally, you can try any of the products listed at the end of this chapter.

Gut flora imbalance issues (see chapter 8) are also likely to flare up with detox overload—so watch for digestive or other symptoms that might be connected to gut flora imbalance (see pages 109–110). This phenomenon occurs because the liver is your major detox organ, but it is also an important part of the immune system. Detoxing causes your liver to have to work harder. If your liver is also already stressed from too many toxins or some other reason, it may be temporarily weaker, and thus your immune system may also end up temporarily weakened. The result is opportunistic parasites like *Candida* yeast and unhealthy bacteria suddenly increasing, and the symptoms associated with that issue suddenly worsening.

People who already have health issues are much more likely to have this type of scenario develop because their immune systems and liver are likely already more stressed and weakened. (Remember that almost all chronic health issues are linked to chronic inflammation, which means a stressed immune system. Since our liver is an important part of our immune system, there is a good chance that it is also stressed.) If you experience increased symptoms with vibration, I recommend assuming that you might have done too much WBV. Stop vibrating and check out the detox products below and the chapter on gut flora. When you feel better, you can start up again—using less vibration.

Detox Support Products

- **Modified citrus pectin** (PectaSol brand recommended): This comes in powder or capsule form, so take one scoop (or six capsules) once a day. This is a great product that is absorbed into your bloodstream and goes everywhere in your body. PectaSol also will absorb only toxins, including heavy metals that have been released into your bloodstream. It can be taken with or without food.

- **ProtoClear** (by Protocol for Life Balance): This is an excellent liver-supporting and detoxing nutritional powder that combines 50+ detox support vitamins, nutrients, herbs, and other products including PectaSol. Take one scoop once a day. It is available on Amazon.

- **Homeopathics:** Consult with a homeopath (see pages 215–216 for help finding a homeopath) for your specific situation. Sometimes additional products and/or homeopathics are needed to resolve a situation.

- **Green smoothies:** You can buy "super greens" powder mixes that combine detoxing and supportive herbs, algae, sprouted grasses, veggies, antioxidant berries and spices, and more. Drink these powders by themselves or add to your regular smoothie. Look for a green drink supplement that contains many different products. Part of the benefit is just that you are getting so many nutrients. Ideally, these ingredients should be organically grown, non-GMO, and processed carefully to preserve nutrients. A high-quality powdered product should also not contain unhealthy additives or common triggers such as wheat, corn, and cane sugar.

- **Activated charcoal:** This product can sometimes be helpful, particularly for localized digestive symptoms, but be sure to take it on an empty stomach (one hour before food or two hours after food) and for not more than a few days because it will absorb nutrients as well as toxins. Take two capsules three times a day.

Heavy Metals

Heavy metals, such as mercury, lead, aluminum, arsenic, and cadmium are particularly dangerous and inflammatory toxins. They are unfortunately easily encountered in modern life and not easily removed from your body. They are found in certain foods (some seafood, as mentioned above), cookware, cosmetics and personal care products, dental fillings, pesticides, old paint, cigarette smoke, polluted air, industrial processes, and more.

If you are over the age of fifty and have been living a typical modern life, there is a good chance you have toxic levels of heavy metals in your body and would benefit from a program to remove them.

Your body stores heavy metals in fat cells, where they are isolated from more vulnerable and critical tissues, but they are hard to remove there. WBV alone will probably not be enough to remove heavy metals, but there are products that can be used to "chelate" or pull these toxins out of your body. A natural health doctor can work with you to assess your situation and remove heavy metals.

You can check your level of heavy metal toxicity with online hair analysis. This is an excellent method to assess long-term low-level exposure (the most common type), as heavy metals and other toxins build up over time in hair. Industrial accidents cause sudden high-level exposures to toxins and show up in blood tests, while long-term exposure will often not show up in blood tests.

If your hair analysis test comes back with elevated levels of heavy metals, be sure to contact your doctor, as heavy metal poisoning can be serious. Because heavy metals are so damaging, they are tricky to deal with. You may need to first heal your gut and calm inflammation with the other methods in this book, so that your body is strong and healthy enough to tolerate chelation.

Chelation uses amino acid products such as EDTA, DMSA, or DMSO to bind with and effectively pull heavy metals out of your body.[3] Your doctor can administer intravenous chelation, or you can use chelating suppositories at home with your doctor's guidance. Be sure to support your body during this process with glutathione and other liver-protective antioxidants. EDTA plus glutathione suppositories are ideal; they are much less expensive than intravenous chelation, and they deliver small doses of EDTA, making this form of chelation gentler and safer. Orally ingested chelation is less effective due to the destruction of the chelation agents by stomach acid.

Heavy Metal Detoxification

EDTA plus glutathione suppositories: This product can provide an effective, safe, and inexpensive heavy metal detox (please consult with a doctor before use). The brand I recommend is Detoxamin. Note that this brand has different strength EDTA products available; unless otherwise advised by a doctor, get the lowest strength version. Remember that slow and gentle is good.

Chapter 10

Exercise

Exercise has long been known to be critical for health, protecting you from everything from heart disease, obesity, diabetes, and depression to practically every other chronic disease. Exercise also lowers chronic inflammation levels—no wonder it protects you from so many illnesses. Whole body vibration (WBV) is exercise, but it is more like weightlifting than aerobic exercise, which is also important. WBV can, however, help you get going on an aerobic exercise program that has numerous benefits such as increased energy, strength, improved mood, and decreased pain. Adding one short aerobic exercise session each day will increase the anti-inflammation effects of your WBV program, bringing you additional healing benefits.

Even a small amount of aerobic exercise can go a long way. According to a recent study at the University of California, San Diego School of Medicine, a single twenty-minute session of moderate exercise can have anti-inflammatory effects on your immune system.[1] With those kinds of results, imagine what a daily twenty-minute walk around the block could do for you! Hundreds of studies have shown that exercise has beneficial effects on the immune system and alleviates chronic inflammation.

WBV can be used for exercise in a wide range of intensities, from very gentle (where you are just standing on the machine) to the intense workouts (see chapter 13) that highly trained athletes engage in. If you have chronic inflammation, you should start gently to keep stress levels down and give your body a chance to heal; start with just one minute of WBV at the lowest speed setting and build up slowly (see chapter 13). Even a tiny amount of WBV can lead to rapid improvements in strength, energy, mobility and balance, pain levels, and mood—all of which makes it easier to add other exercise. As your inflammation and pain levels decrease, you can increase the time and intensity of your aerobic exercise and your WBV workout, getting stronger and healthier all the time.

You can also use WBV for stretching and as a warm-up before working out; it is wonderfully effective for loosening up, and it can increase your athletic performance by heightening your senses, boosting hormones and mood, and giving you extra energy. WBV also raises levels of human growth hormone, which will help you recover from all types of exercise faster, and you can use WBV after a workout to relax with targeted massage positions.

Exercise Is a Fountain of Youth

There are many proven benefits to exercise. The body is designed for physical activity, and it thrives on it. For example,

> ## TESTIMONIAL
>
> **Using my vibration plate feels like a mini vacation; I started slow, with just a few minutes, and I enjoy it; it relaxes me, and my body feels happy. At night, the body pain I had in bed is gone and there is a real satisfaction in sleeping that I have not had for years. I am more in tune and listening to my body, and I have much more courage and the willpower to start a physical activity like biking. This is encouraging; I am excited to see how my health continues to improve.**
>
> **I have also noticed that the varicose veins on my leg are getting much better. They have stopped bulging out and seem to be slowly fading away. This is exciting, as I was not expecting to improve this issue with the vibration. I feel like so many options are opening to me, with a future that I was not expecting. Thank you so much, Becky!**
>
> —Giuseppe Pallotta, age 52

exercise increases your circulation, bringing essential nutrients and oxygen to every part of your body, including your brain, and removing waste products. Amping up this process helps every cell and organ in your body to function at a higher level. And, just by exercising, you increase your body's ability to drive the circulatory system. Your heart, which pumps blood through the arteries on its outgoing journey, becomes stronger. Exercising builds more muscle, which in turn massages the veins in the gentler but essential pumping action that moves the blood on its return trip to the heart. Exercise, whether in a more traditional form or with WBV, is also critical to maintaining muscle tone, bone density, and a healthy weight.

The body is designed for physical activity, and it thrives on it.

Just as important as the effects on your body, exercise helps your brain, protecting you from inflammation-related diseases such as Alzheimer's, Parkinson's, and multiple sclerosis. Exercise is also effective for alleviating stress, a proven inflammation-reducing strategy. Cortisol, a major stress hormone, goes down, and mental health improves. Exercise increases the levels of natural chemicals in your brain called neurotransmitters—an effect that will raise your spirits, energize you, and help your brain to function better. Exercise has also been shown to increase the number of neurons and neural connections in your brain. These are important components of intelligence, so you may actually be getting smarter as you exercise.

How Much and What Type of Exercise?

Like with WBV, to reduce inflammation with any exercise, start gently and increase slowly. Too much exercise can raise stress and inflammation in your body. How much is too much depends on your current level of health and fitness. If you have not been exercising, and are older and/or dealing with health issues, you will need to start more gently than a younger person who gets more exercise in their daily life.

Most importantly, find some type of exercise that works for you—something you enjoy and that works for your body. This will go a long way toward keeping your exercise program going long term. You can walk, bike, dance, swim, do yoga or tai chi—whatever makes you happy.

Start with an amount that pushes you a little beyond your comfort zone but not into pain. Listen to your body. Try to get your heart rate up, your breathing deeper, and feel your muscles working, but slow down or stop if you are feeling pain. In the beginning, aim for at least twenty minutes four to five times a week; start with less if you need to.

As you begin to feel better, increase the length of your workout. As a goal, try to work up to thirty to sixty minutes of vigorous exercise at least three to four times a week. Longer and more intense exercise like this will give you the beta-endorphin "runner's high" and higher levels of other feel-good neurotransmitters.

Try adding interval training to your exercise program. Alternating bursts of more intense effort followed by lower intensity recovery periods has been shown to multiply the benefits of exercise.[2] This is easy—try five to ten cycles of thirty-second bursts of intense effort, alternating with one to two minutes of less intense effort. For example, while walking, try speeding up for short distances, then relaxing and checking out the view with a slower pace for a few minutes, then put on the steam again! Keep this alternating pattern going for ten to fifteen minutes, and you will have amplified the effects of your workout, giving you the benefits of a considerably longer walk.

Try combining stress reduction methods (see chapter 11) with your exercise. For example, being in nature is a well-known stress reducer, so if you walk or bike outside with interval training, you will be getting the benefits of amped up exercise plus nature at the same time.

Chapter 11

Meditation, Yoga, and Other Therapies to Reduce Stress

Reducing the constant stress of modern life can be a powerful method for decreasing inflammation and moving the mind and body into a calmer state where they can focus on healing and repair. Hundreds, if not thousands, of studies have demonstrated the connection between lower stress and improved health and lower inflammation. Whole body vibration has impressive antistress and relaxation effects; combining it with other de-stressing methods will create even greater synergistic effects. Try adapting yoga, tai chi, or any other relaxation method so that you can do it while on your vibration machine. This will give you a synergistic effect increasing the power of both.

Natural De-Stressing Methods

Acupuncture: Acupuncture has a long history of relieving pain and lowering stress. This can be a very helpful mode of healing to add to your program. For more information and resources, see www.nccaom.org.

Whole body vibration has powerful antistress and relaxation effects; combining it with other de-stressing methods will create even greater synergistic effects.

Art, music, and dance: Express yourself with an art form or enjoy beautiful, calming and/or inspiring music, art, and dance. Studies show that just thirty minutes of listening to music can drop cortisol levels. Art is a well-known therapeutic mode of expression and communication. And dancing to your favorite songs can relieve stress and give you exercise at the same time.

Breathing: There are remarkable benefits reported from focused breathing techniques. Slow, measured breathing can be relaxing and bring relief from many conditions, including immune system and inflammatory conditions.[1] There are many resources online for breathing exercises and methods; for example, https://www.healthline.com/health/breathing-exercise#pursed-lip-breathing. James Nestor's book *Breath: The New Science of a Lost Art* is a fascinating look at the science and benefits of breathing.

Chiropractic: Some back issues are contraindications for WBV, such as acute herniated or bulging disks. Chiropractic care can be very helpful for this type of back issue, as well as other back pain and body issues. Chiropractic can be a great addition to your health program, and when an acute disc issue is better, then you can add in WBV.

Conversation and connection: We all need connection—it is a basic element of psychological health. Chatting with friends or family can help reduce stress. In-person connections with friends and family is ideal. If you can't do that, call and talk on the phone or video chat with Zoom, Skype, Facebook messenger, or WhatsApp. Need more connections? Join a group interested in activities you enjoy: dancing, music, knitting, cats, computer games—there's a group for every imaginable activity and interest. For example, Google Meetup is an international online group that facilitates finding others with common interests.

Energy exercises: Yoga, tai chi, and qigong are energy exercise systems. Energy exercises have been developed over the ages by numerous different cultures. The most important thing is to incorporate a practice of movement and relaxation into your life and do it regularly. Adapt as needed to try these exercises on a vibrating plate for an extra blast of energy and relaxation.

Homeopathy: Homeopathy is a form of energy medicine with a two hundred-year history of lowering inflammation and healing health issues[2]—a hidden jewel in the medical world. Homeopathy uses resonating energy waves to help release stress and negative thoughts and emotions. Because of the close mind/body connection, this can lead to body-wide relief from health issues.

Hot tubs, jacuzzi, whirlpools, saunas: Relax with heat and water. For an extra stimulating boost, follow your heat therapy with a quick dip in cold water.

Meditation and prayer: Meditation and other focusing methods have been used for centuries to help de-stress and quiet the static of a busy mind and to connect with a higher power. There are many meditation methods in books, online, and through courses. You can simply sit and focus on your breathing or listen to guided meditations or meditate in groups. There is something for everybody, and what works for someone else may not work for you, so try some different methods and use them as best fits you. Check online and in the Suggested Reading section for books and CDs to get you started.

Nature: There are now over one thousand studies looking into the health effects of spending time in nature. The evidence is conlcusive that time spent in nature, as long as you feel safe, results in lower blood pressure and stress hormone levels, reduced nervous system arousal, enhanced immune system function, increased self-esteem, reduced anxiety, and improved mood.[3] As a Yale University paper on the subject put it, these studies "point in one direction: Nature is not only nice to have, but it's a have-to-have for physical health and cognitive functioning."[4]

There are numerous factors that contribute to the health effects of nature, including sunlight, increased oxygen and fresh air, peace, beauty, and perspective—perhaps also beneficial effects from vibrations and wavelengths received from the multitude of natural sources you are exposed to outdoors.

Sunlight increases the production of vitamin D—which is essential for the production of serotonin, as well as a healthy immune system and bones. Sunlight also helps to control the levels of melatonin, a hormone that affects our sleep and wake cycles. And sleep, of course, is critical to physical as well as mental health.

The increase in oxygen from breathing fresh air will also help your body and immune system to function properly. Every cell in your body and brain requires oxygen, just as a fire cannot burn without oxygen, your cells depend on oxygen to burn fuel and create energy to do their jobs—including to heal your body and lower inflammation. So, get outside and enjoy! As John Denver put it, "Sunshine on my shoulders makes me happy!"

Chapter 12

Choosing a Whole Body Vibration Machine

Over the last twenty years, I have used and sold a lot of different vibration machines. I have seen, with myself and from working with hundreds of clients, that the type of machine you use, especially with seniors and others with health challenges, is critical to the success of whole body vibration. Since problems can develop from using the wrong machine (see below), I am careful about which whole body vibration machines I use and recommend. Eventually, using my knowledge and experience, I designed and developed my own machines to ensure that I can supply the best type of machines to my clients and customers.

With the increasing popularity of whole body vibration, there has been an surge of interest in making and selling vibration machines, resulting in a plethora of confusing promotional information. I can only recommend with complete confidence my own machines and others that you will find on my website.

For your convenience, my machines are listed below. If you want to understand the field and options for other types of machines, more information about these subjects follows; but be prepared, it is a jungle of information. My machines are available on my website and on Amazon. Check my website (BCVibrantHealth.com) for the latest information.

The most important information for many people is that you don't need to spend a great deal of money to get enormous benefit. There is a huge range of machines, and you can get an effective and therapeutic device for less than a gym membership and much less than what you might spend on health care. Considering all the benefits to your health, you will likely end up saving a great deal of money.

Currently, there are three Vibrant Health machines. The g-force for my machines is proprietary information, which is why I don't list amplitudes and g-forces. My machines are designed to heal, but exactly what goes into creating this vibration is complicated, and my formula is restricted. There are many factors that go into creating this best type of vibration; other companies cannot copy my machines, as they are not aware of what is needed. My machines are based on twenty years of experience trying many machines and studying the effects, particularly for people with chronic health issues. My results—which you can see in appendix 1, on my website, and in my books—are your assurance that my machines will provide you with what you need. I cannot vouch for other companies' machines.

1. **Vibrant Health Power 1000:** Vibrant Health's most popular model, this machine delivers a vibration powerful

enough to give you an intense workout, but it is still gentle enough to be very safe and easy to use. This machine is designed for people of all ages. It is especially ideal for children, busy adults, baby boomers, and seniors. It is the perfect machine for optimizing both physical and mental health with a carefully designed, perfectly synchronized, smooth vibration. It will deliver a challenging workout and/or deep massage and stretching for tight muscles, plus the best vibration for brain function and brain wave synchronization. Standing upright on this plate, you will feel the vibration travel through your entire body and up into your head—but don't worry, it feels good and is not bad for you!

The vertical vibration motion of this machine feels like a powerful cheetah purring. Because this motion is so smooth, the average person, with normal balance, will not need a handle to hold on to. If you do have balance issues, you can buy an optional tower and handle to go with the machine, use a separate balance bar, or put the vibration plate next to something else to hold on to. There are also two kinds of straps for use with different arm exercise positions: stretchy and non-stretchy.

Frequency range: 26–45 Hz
Cost: $999
BCVibrantHealth.com
Amazon: Search for "BC Vibrant Health Power 1000"
Or use this link: https://www.amazon.com/gp/product/B07D3BZRS8

2. **VIBRANT HEALTH GENTLE 500:** This machine provides the best type of vibration—but the amplitude of the motion is less than that of the Vibrant Health Power 1000, making this machine more suited to more fragile people. This gentle machine is ideal for those on a budget or with age and/or health issues that make them more sensitive.

When you stand on this vertical vibration machine, it produces a motion similar in sensation to a cat purring; you will feel the vibration travel up your body into your legs. You can get vibration into other parts of your body by sitting on the machine or doing exercises where your hands are on the machine, such as push-ups.

There is a tower with the control panel right in front of you and a handle to hold on to for people with balance issues.

> Frequency range: 30–45 Hz
> Cost: $499
> BCVibrantHealth.com
> Amazon: Search for "Becky Chambers Vibrant Health Gentle 500"
> Or use this link: https://www.amazon.com/dp/B07D3D172S?

3. **VIBRANT HEALTH FOOT VIBRATING MASSAGE SHAKER:** Foot vibration machines are a new option for people who are fragile and older or not yet ready to invest in a bigger, more expensive machine but still want to dip their feet into vibration technology. These devices are lightweight, small, inexpensive, and easy—you just sit on a chair next to the device and put your

feet on it or lie on the ground and rest your arms or legs on it. As they are smaller and lighter weight, you can also take them with you when you travel.

Automatic foot and leg movements trigger muscle fibers to tighten and relax and nerves to shoot signals to your brain waking it up. Circulation increases, bringing nutrients and oxygen to your tissues, removing waste products. They are also good for lymphatic drainage and detoxification, as your leg and foot muscle fibers massage and move toxins through your lymphatic system.

The direction of motion is vertical, but it is a different system that allows the heels of your feet to move more than your toes, causing a shaking motion that gives your leg muscles movement as well as vibration. Since you cannot stand or put much weight on these devices, the more intensive, full-body exercise options that are available with larger vibration machines are not possible.

Other companies also offer foot vibrating devices. Be careful not to get a device that delivers only massage and not vibration. They may feel good, but they won't deliver the same benefits.

> 3 vibration speeds plus massage
> Cost: $149
> Available through BCVibrantHealth.com

Double-Motor Vibration Machines

The first whole body vibration machines were developed for Olympic athletes. To achieve greater power, thus a greater workout effect, these machines had two motors in them. Many machines made and sold now continue to use this technology and still have two motors in them. But most of us are not Olympic athletes or football players, and, especially if you are dealing with health issues, your body and mind will need a different approach.

Additionally, two motors can send an unsynchronized message into your body, which can have a desynchronizing effect on your nervous system and energy field and potentially disrupt a healthy state of brain synchronization. I do not recommend this type of machine for anyone. As any engineer can attest, it is impossible to completely synchronize two motors.

Brain synchronization is the simultaneous, in-phase firing of brain cells. These combined signals generate electromagnetic brain waves, which can be measured by electroencephalography (EEG) and magnetic resonance imaging (MRI). Brain synchronization has been linked to increases in creativity, memory, learning, problem solving, and intuition, as well as to improvements for depression, anxiety, and ADHD.[xvi] While people cannot detect the millisecond lack of synchronization on a double-motor vibration machine at a conscious level, your nervous system and energy fields are extremely sensitive, and, on a deeper, unconscious level, they will be picking up this discordant effect.

Health effects from desynchronization can be difficult to recognize and detect, especially in strong, healthy people. Since the athletes who typically use this type of machine have such strong overall health, this side effect may go unnoticed for years. By the time trouble begins to develop (and since it involves the nervous

---

[xvi]There have been many studies to back these claims. Please see the "Brain Synchronization" section under Additional Research Studies at the back of the book.

system and brain, which controls your entire body, it can show up as any type of problem), these users have seen so many positive effects that they do not suspect they may be using the wrong sort of vibration machine.

But with older and otherwise more sensitive or fragile people, this effect can be seen much more quickly and dramatically. I believe this may be part of the explanation for why some research on WBV with older people and those with health issues has not been as good as was hoped for and expected based on early research with animals and healthy young athletes.

My Experience with a Double-Motor Machine

For me, as the sensitive canary in the mine, problems quickly became clear. After my first six months with one of these double-motor machines, during which I did see improvements and became stronger than I had been in many years, my health suddenly deteriorated. I experienced a sudden and mysterious downturn and had such severe muscle weakness that I could not make it up the stairs or even across the room (this after having improved from years of debilitating health issues to climbing Mt. Washington only two weeks earlier).

My allergies, chemical sensitivities, multiple infections, digestive distress, and nervous-system problems also all returned. It seemed to be linked to the vibration, somehow, as I would get much worse after the slightest amount, but what exactly about the vibration was bothering me was difficult to determine.

Dr. DeOrio, an early expert in WBV[1] and my doctor at that time, theorized that it was a desynchronization effect from the double-motor machine that was causing my sudden downturn. After much trial and error, and eventually switching to a single-motor machine, it became clear that he was correct; only desynchronizing vibration was causing problems, not single-motor vertical vibration, which provides a fully synchronized signal to one's nervous system. I have now been exclusively using single-motor vertical vibration machines for fifteen years without a problem.

In fact, the proper type of vibration machine—vibration that sends a gentle and fully synchronized signal into my brain—aided me in my recovery. With this type of machine, I eventually fully recovered and have since then not only healed most of my long-standing health issues but also reached greater heights of achievement and happiness than I ever thought possible—mentally and physically!

Different Models and Makes

There are many companies now selling vibration machines, and some machines are sold by many different distributors under different names, sometimes for widely varying prices; it can be hard to know exactly what type of vibration you are buying. There are also different terms used for important features of vibration machines, and sometimes the same word is used to refer to opposite things. I will try to clarify, but because of rampant misleading marketing, this task is difficult.

Vibration machines were first developed (and are still best known) for their ability to create an intense workout. Many WBV-machine companies have the football-player mindset that the more power the better. Thus, many of the best-selling machines, and most of the machines you will find in health clubs and sports centers, are of the double-motor variety or produce a large amplitude and g-force with a wilder type of motion called "oscillation" (see below). Beyond this issue, there are several other variables to consider: direction of movement, power (g-force), amplitudes, frequencies, durability, and cost.

Direction of Movement

VERTICAL VIBRATION MOTION

There are two major types of motion for vibration plates. Vertical (or linear) motion machines vibrate mostly up and down. This is the type of machine that I recommend for most people. Unfortunately, some companies are now misleadingly renaming other motions with this vertical vibration term—to gain market share. I have seen completely different motions, such as oscillation (see below), described as vertical vibration.

When the vertical vibration is actually a *true* vertical vibration, in which the entire plate moves in a uniform motion directly up and down and the vibration is produced with only one motor, this will provide a completely synchronized movement and message to your system. This motion is also the most stabilizing for your structural system. This is the type of motion I use in my machines.

Further confusion is created by variations of this first basic type of motion being produced by different motor configurations, including the double-motor machines mentioned earlier.

The different motor types confer small amounts of horizontal motion and circular movement to the plate, along with the predominantly vertical motion. To seem different (and better), companies come up with novel names, such as three-dimensional, horizontal, spiral, circular, tri-planar, triangular, tri-phasic, multi-dimensional, omniflex, and piston. All these terms are describing basically the same type of motion.

> *When the vertical vibration is actually a true vertical vibration, . . . this will provide a completely synchronized movement and message to your system.*

There is also a great variation in amplitudes, g-force, durability, and cost with these machines. The intensity of your vibration workout depends on the power, or gravitational force (g-force), of the vibration—a factor that takes into account the amplitude and frequency of the machine and the weight (your own weight) that your muscles must hold against the vibration. As amplitudes, frequency, and your weight can vary greatly, there is great flexibility in the intensity of your workout.

To get a sense of what I mean by g-force, imagine putting your hand on a purring cat versus holding a jackhammer—these are very different experiences because of the different amplitudes and weights. A jackhammer's amplitude of vibration, and its weight, are much greater than those of a hand resting on a purring cat, so even though the frequencies of these vibrations are similar, the total g-force, and therefore effect, is greater for the jackhammer.

Frequency ranges with vertical vibration machines are typically about 20–50 Hz—much higher than frequencies found in oscillation motion machines (0–20 Hz[xvii]). This is because the motion of a vertical vibration machine is so much smoother that it can run much faster without a problem—a motion that is somewhat similar to that of a cat purring, though it can range from a gentle pussy cat to a cheetah's purr to a motion perhaps more like a giant, prehistoric saber-toothed cat's purr (assuming giant, prehistoric saber-toothed cats purred). At the upper end of this range is the potentially disruptive, and not recommended, vibration of a double-motor machine.

Oscillation Vibration Motion

A second major type of vibration machine utilizes oscillation across a fulcrum in the middle of the plate, so that the plate rises and falls on either side like a child's seesaw. This motion is called oscillation, pivotal, or teeter-totter, and it is quite popular; probably because you can achieve a large amount of motion and a high g-force for a low cost. However, the speed is much slower than vertical vibration and the movement much wilder, so the effect is quite different.[xviii]

Oscillation vibration machines have high maximum amplitudes but low frequencies, in contrast to true vertical vibration machines, which have lower amplitudes and high frequencies.

[xvii]To hide this lower range of frequencies because potential customers are searching for higher speeds, many oscillation machine companies arbitrarily label the speed range without the Hz designation. So, the speeds may be listed as 1–60, but really go up to only 20 Hz.

[xviii]Thus, these companies can claim that their vibration machines have the highly sought-after characteristics of high amplitude and g-force without spending the money to produce the powerful, true vertical vibration machines.

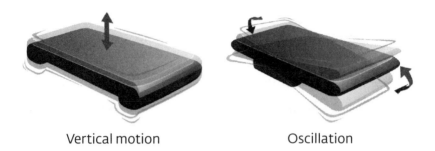

Vertical motion   Oscillation

Oscillation vibration machines need to run slower because the motion would be too wild if the speed was high at the same time as the amplitude of motion—remember that this motion is similar to that of a seesaw, with a large movement at each end of the plate and very little movement in the center of the plate. These machines can provide power and high g-forces for less cost. But the wilder motion caused by essentially having a foot on each end of a rapidly moving seesaw can be destabilizing for your musculoskeletal system and create more stress for body and mind.

For ease of use and total health, I recommend a single-motor, vertical vibration machine with its perfect synchronization and smooth motion. While I believe that people of any age should avoid machines that create stress and/or destabilization, I feel it is extra important for older people and anyone whose health, including brain health, is more vulnerable.

A second major type of vibration machine utilizes oscillation across a fulcrum in the middle of the plate, so that the plate rises and falls on either side like a child's seesaw.

Hybrid-Motion Machines

There are now machines that have multiple types of motion controlled by multiple motors within one device. They can have up to three motors in them with three different types of motion, the two described above and a motion they label "horizontal" that has not been studied much, if at all, though health claims are still made. They also often have the option of operating multiple motions at one time. *Don't do that!* Never combine different types of motion, as this could lead to the desynchronizing effects described earlier.

These companies are trying to give you every possibility in one machine because they don't know what is best, and they want you to buy their machine. Typically, these machines give you a little bit of everything but not enough (too low an amplitude and g-force) of the best, vertical type of vibration.

If you want vibration for healing, hybrid machines are not the best choice. I cannot recommend confusing the vibrational message going into your body, any more than an acupuncturist would put needles randomly all over your body.

I believe that the clarity of the electromagnetic signal from a single-motor, vertical vibration machine contributes to the superior results that I achieve.

Oscillation and other types of vibration are not more effective in the long run for total health, and do not provide as coherent, clear, and smooth a signal for the nervous system as single-motor vertical vibration. For these reasons I only recommend single-motor, vertical vibration.

SONIC VIBRATION

The final type of machine is one in which a true vertical vibration motion is generated by sonic (sound) waves. No actual sound is produced by these machines; the term "sonic" is used here to describe a sound wave–type of mechanism that produces a vertical movement, not a sound. These machines typically create smooth and synchronized vibrations with a large range of amplitudes as well as frequencies, but the cost is also very high ($3,000 to $10,000) without significant additional benefits for the average user.

Remember, a greater amplitude and g-force does not mean better! The machines I most often recommend are $500 to $1,000.

Intense exercise is only one of many benefits you can get from vibration. For many people, if they try to work out too intensely with vibration at the beginning, they will end up increasing inflammation and feeling worse instead of better because of too much stress and detoxing. Be patient! Remember that you can get exercise many ways. The workout effect is not the only benefit, and it is not what makes vibration so unique. Muscle strength, toning, and weight loss are only the tip of the iceberg when it comes to vibration's benefits.

Gravitational (g) Force, Amplitude, and Frequency

The power of a machine (g-force) is determined by the amplitude (the distance the plate moves), the frequency (the rate or speed of vibration), and the weight of the person on the plate. The greater the amplitude, the frequency, and the weight, the greater the g-force. Again, imagine putting your hand on a purring cat versus holding a jackhammer—these are very different experiences because of the different amplitudes and weights involved, even though the frequencies of vibration are similar. G-force is a common way people compare machines, though it is not an exact method, as people's weights vary significantly, and weight is a component for determining g-force.

Changing the amplitude dramatically changes the g-force; with a low-amplitude vibration feeling like the purring cat versus high-amplitude machines that can rattle your body with their more jackhammer-type vibration. To change the amplitude, one often needs to change machines.

G-force and amplitude have become a hot topic, with many consumers searching for high numbers. This market pressure has led to some companies artificially inflating g-force and amplitude numbers. It is like women's dress sizes—we get bigger, but dress sizes stay the same or go down . . . because that is what we want!

In response to people wanting high-amplitude (high-power) machines and making buying decisions based on this factor, some companies use a peak-to-peak measurement of amplitude versus the standard centerline-to-peak amplitude measurement (see diagram on next page). Using the peak-to-peak-measurement method produces amplitudes twice as big as the centerline method, without actually changing the true vibration. Other companies deal with this issue by not giving amplitude information at all. When amplitude information is given, there is no explanation or consensus as to which measurement is being referenced.

Double-motor, vertical-motion machines can deliver high amplitudes, frequencies, and g-forces, but (as I noted earlier) I don't recommend these machines, and they are expensive, ranging from $3,500 to $10,000. Oscillating motion machines have even higher amplitudes, but since the motion is so wild, the frequency is much lower. The resulting maximum g-forces can go quite high with these machines, though not as high as the maximum g-forces in double-motor, vertical vibration machines.

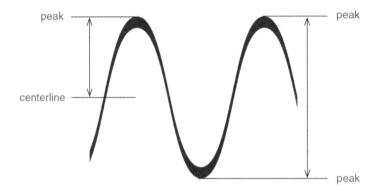

Most machines have a wide range of frequency (speed) settings. Vertical vibration machines have settings ranging around 20–50 Hz (vibrations per second). Oscillation machines typically have lower frequency ranges (often 1–20 Hz). Many, maybe most, oscillation machine manufacturers obfuscate their low speeds by creating an arbitrary numerical scale—so, though their machine's maximum frequency setting might be only 20 Hz, that setting might be called 60 or even 100 in their speed settings.

Much effort has gone into figuring out which frequencies, types of motion, and positions on the machine are the best for losing weight and cellulite, increasing bone density and muscle strength, lymph drainage, et cetera. My experience is that focusing on exactly what frequency is the best for achieving certain effects is a moot point for beginners. By far the most important issue, when beginning, is to start at a low frequency and increase slowly so that you lower inflammation and stress, allowing your body and mind to heal itself.

However, as you become able to tolerate the higher frequencies, these questions become more important, and higher settings are beneficial and do have more powerful effects (see page 164 for more details). *Always go slowly,* or you may end up disappointed and stop entirely! My book *Whole Body Vibration for Seniors* also has physical therapy guidelines and recommendations for specific health issues. And remember that even gentle vibration will be affecting your whole body and giving you anti-inflammatory effects. So, no matter what frequency or amplitude of a single-motor, vertical vibration machine you use, as long as you also do not do too much and overstress your body, you will be on your way to lowering inflammation and achieving the desired results.

Regarding which type of motion is best, as I have explained, I believe the smooth but powerful motion of a mid-range amplitude, vertical vibration machine is usually best. Other machines may provide a bigger workout or specific effect (such as lymphatic drainage), but the stress of these machines on your body and brain may interfere with healing your whole system. Quick-fix effects like these pale in comparison to the long-term health benefits of a gentler approach and optimizing WBV for the brain, especially for people with health issues.

For very sensitive, older, or ill people, the best choice may be a very low amplitude vertical vibration machine or a foot vibration device. See the machine comparison section that follows for options.

Durability

This depends on the quality of construction. Plastic parts are not as durable as steel, but for low-cost, low–g-force machines, plastic can be a reasonable option. Larger, more powerful machines are usually made of steel and can weigh quite a lot. Many machines are made overseas and shipped to the US. Quality can vary widely, so be sure to check the warranty terms and weight limits for users. Generally, the higher the g-force and amplitude of a machine, the larger, heavier, and more expensive it is likely to be. This is because the motor must be more powerful to generate the greater amplitude, and since vibration tends to shake things apart, the machine must be built to withstand increasing force.

Cost

There is an enormous range in the cost of machines. You can spend anywhere from $150 for a small foot vibration device, to $200 for an inexpensive, cheaply made oscillation or vertical vibration machine, to $13,000 for some sonic vibration machines, and everything in between. The cost depends on many factors, including the type of machine and amount of power, the quality of construction, availability of knowledgeable customer support, demand, and the marketing strategy—the same machine made in Asia is selling in different places for a tenfold difference in price. Note, when checking out machines, how exactly the same some supposedly different machines look. On the other hand, there are also copycat machines for sale; inferior, cheaply made machines that have been carefully designed to look like an expensive one—it is the Wild West out there.

Below is a comparison of different companies making and selling machines. My highest recommendation is single-motor, vertical vibration, but I can only vouch for the machines that you will find on my website. My machines are specially formulated to meet all of the requirements my many years of experience have shown to be critical for the best results. I cannot recommend other machines as I cannot be sure exactly how they are made. In the comparisons below, I will outline the features of my machines, as well as, to the best of my ability, the basic features of a large selection of the many other machines on the market. As new machines are always coming on the market, I will post and update this information on my website.

Vibration Machines Comparisons

This information was accurate as of late 2021. See Becky's Vibrant Health website (BCVibrantHealth.com) for the latest updates.

Single-Motor, Relatively Gentle, Vertical Vibration Machines (Recommended)

Vibrant Health machines: See beginning of this chapter for complete details.

VibePlate: Has eight different models with different-sized plates.
>Maximum amplitude: 2 mm (centerline-to-peak measurement)
>Frequency range: 10–60 Hz
>Cost: ranges from $1,195 to $6,995

Bulletproof: One model only.
>Maximum amplitude: listed as 4 mm on their website—with a note that this is a **peak-to-peak** measurement. More standard **centerline-to-peak amplitude would be 2 mm.**
>Frequency: 30 Hz (no variability)
>Cost: $1,495

Single-Motor, Very Gentle, Low-Amplitude, Vertical Vibration (Recommended)

These machines are very gentle and have low amplitudes (less than 1 mm) and low gravitational forces (0.3–0.4 g). **They are not very effective for bone building and workouts, but they are very safe and a good alternative when a person cannot tolerate the stronger vibrations of the mid-level machines above.**

Juvent: There are two models.
>Frequency range: 32–37 Hz
>Cost: ranges from $3,400 to $5,200

Marodyne: There is one model, the Marodyne LIVmd.
>Frequency: 30 Hz (no variability)
>Cost: about $2,000

Sonic Vibration Machines (Recommended)

SonicLife: There are four models of Sonix vibration machines.
> Frequency ranges: 4–30 Hz for the least expensive model; 3–70 Hz for the most expensive model
> Cost: ranges from $2,995 to $9,995

Double-Motor and Double-Motion Vibration Machines (Not Recommended)

The motion is called by numerous different names, often reflecting complicated systems (in which more than one direction and type of movement can operate at the same time) and/or the very forceful nature of this type of machine: triplaner, spiral, circular, three-dimensional, horizontal, triangular, triphasic, multidimensional, omniflex, and piston. Double-motion machines will also include oscillation motion. Generally, for the triplaner type of motion, amplitudes range from 3–6 mm, frequencies ranges are 20–50 Hz, and maximum g-forces are 6–15 g. Oscillation motion modes have amplitudes of 1–12 mm, frequencies of 1–20 Hz, and maximum g-forces up to 8 g.

PowerPlate: There are numerous triplaner, double-motor models. Possibly PowerPlate now also makes a single-motor machine, but this is hard to determine for sure, as they do not post or discuss this information on their website.
> Cost: ranges from $1,495 to $12,995

DKN: They have four triplaner models.
> Cost: ranges from $2,499 to $4,699

Vmax: There are numerous different models (including Vmax, Pulser, Trio, ProDuo, Elite, Q2, Q5), most of which can run with both types of motion.

Cost: ranges from $1,248 to $4,699

IVibration: There is one model with multiple types of vibration produced concurrently.

Cost: $1,695

Tectonic: They have three models, two of which are double motion, and one is oscillation motion only.

Cost: ranges from $1,795 to $2,899

TriFlex: This is similar to some Vmax models, running with both types of motion, but is less expensive.

LifePro: They makes numerous models; many, such as the Rumblex, have multiple motors and several types of motion. LifePro also makes oscillation machines (see below).

Oscillation Vibration Machines

This is a popular type of machine (see the long list below of companies making and selling these machines), as you can achieve a high amplitude and g-force for a low price—but this does not mean it is the best type of vibration for you. Also known as pivotal, or teeter-totter, this type of motion can be destabilizing for joints and stressful for the mind and body. (See the earlier section about oscillation machines.) Some of these companies are actually selling the same machines, marketed under different names (notice how similar they look in pictures online). Amplitude ranges are usually 1–10 mm, frequency ranges are usually 1–20 Hz, and maximum g-forces can go up to 8 g. Prices can range from a few hundred dollars to three thousand dollars.

    Bluefin
    Body Trim Fitness
    Confidence Fitness
    Hurdle
    HyperVibe
    iDeer
    LifePro (numerous models—a few have oscillation motion only, many have multiple motors and several types of motion)
    Maketec
    Merax
    Noblerex K1
    Pinty
    Rock Solid
    T-Zone
    VibraPro
    Vmax (models Vmax i25 and Vmax Elite 300)
    Zazz

Chapter 13

Getting Started with Whole Body Vibration

In this chapter, there are daily plans for how to get started, including a beginner's program, and guidelines for more advanced users, including a selection of exercise positions showing the versatility of whole body vibration (WBV). As stated before, WBV can be an intensive workout suitable for elite athletes but can also be adapted for use with people who are not up to exercising yet and need to just focus on lowering inflammation and feeling better. When you are up to exercising, the workout most likely won't make you feel sweaty and exhausted. Until then, the sooner you start your anti-inflammation natural health regimen, the better! First, be sure to check the contraindications listed in appendix 5; also, before starting any therapeutic and/or exercise program, it is advisable to discuss WBV therapy with your physician.

There is a huge variation in how people respond to vibration. If you do not have any health problems and you are just feeling great with WBV, you can increase your time and speed at a much faster pace. A healthy young person might be able to do ten minutes on a powerful machine and feel fine the first time he or she ever uses one. Other people, especially those with health issues, may need months just to get to ten minutes at the lowest speed on a low-power machine. A lot depends on your health and constitution.

For example, I had a sixty-year-old client with chronic fatigue and depression who experienced a dramatic improvement in energy and mood after his first one-minute session at the lowest frequency on a gentle machine. He did not have a long history of health issues, though, and had a robust constitution. He bought that machine and was able to increase to ten minutes at the highest frequency (50 Hz) within a couple of months.

At the other end of the spectrum is me. I have a long history of health problems and am a very sensitive person; so it took me years to get to the highest setting on the same gentle machine, while also taking an impressive number of nutritional products and using other types of natural health therapies.

For improving the general health and well-being for people with inflammation-driven chronic health issues, the goal is to gradually increase the amount of vibration to at least ten minutes per day at a mid-range frequency on a *relatively* gentle or, if necessary, on a *very gentle* vibration machine. This amount of WBV supplies many benefits every day.

If you are having problems of any sort, stop vibrating for a few days and see if you get better. Also check chapter 9 for detox reactions and what to do. When you feel better, try less vibration. Keep in mind that any vibration can have dramatic positive effects, so start slowly. Increase at your own pace—and enjoy!

Whole Body Vibration Training Basics

Goals

- Minimum recommended usage (but work up to this slowly): ten minutes of vibration at a frequency setting of 30–35 Hz each day, but it is not a problem if you miss some days, and don't worry, you will still be getting huge anti-inflammatory and other benefits from lower frequencies. It is great if you can work up to doing twenty minutes per day.

- Maximum recommended usage: twenty to thirty minutes of vibration per day.

Basics

- Once you are feeling up to some exercise, you can target various muscle groups by choosing different positions from the pictures in this book or from the expanded poster of fifty-four positions available on my website and included with the Vibrant Health Power 1000 machine.

- If you have a foot vibration device, you can follow the recommendations in the beginner's program for increasing time and speed. Depending on your health, you may be able to increase more rapidly, as the effect is smaller. You will not be able to use the exercise positions and will remain in a sitting position, though you can get vibration higher in your legs by lying on the floor with your calves or thighs resting on the foot pads of the device, or put your hands on the pads to get vibration into your hands and arms.

- Do each exercise position for thirty seconds to one minute, either holding the position (static, or isometric) or moving in and out of it (dynamic, or kinetic).

- Many benefits are achieved even if you only stand on the machine. In fact, standing upright on the plate is a great position for increasing bone density, as it helps to transmit the vibration throughout your body. So, even if you are too tired to work out, do stand or sit on your plate—relax and vibrate!

- Mid-level speed settings (30–35 Hz) are optimal for massage, stretching, and muscle- and bone-strengthening exercises. Higher speed settings (35–45 Hz) are ideal for brain stimulation. Lower speed settings (26–30 Hz) are perfect for warm ups and cool downs, and for starting out, when you are slowly building up your tolerance for vibration. In the beginning, don't worry about using an optimal speed for working out or for the brain. *The most important thing is to start slowly and just do some vibration!* Remember that *all* vibration on the right kind of machine—and when not doing too much and thus overstressing your body—will help lower inflammation and achieve strengthening, stretching and massage, lymphatic drainage, and other health benefits.

Becky's Slow and Gentle Beginner's Program

These guidelines have been developed particularly with my machines in mind. I cannot vouch for their applicability to other types of machines. If you have a foot vibration device or other vibration machine listed as a recommended "very gentle" machine in my comparison chart (pages 155), you may be able to start with more vibration and increase more quickly than the guidelines here. You might try doubling the time recommendations below.

DAY 1: Stand on your vibration machine (make sure you are using the proper type of machine) for thirty to sixty seconds at the lowest frequency or speed setting. WBV has very powerful effects on every part of your body, so I recommend starting with a very small amount of vibration on the first day to see how you respond. Watch and wait for twenty-four hours before trying any more vibration. As long as you feel the same or better the next day, you can increase the length of time of your next vibration session (see below). Increasing the frequency powerfully intensifies the experience, so first increase the length of time you are on the machine, getting up to ten minutes at the same frequency setting, before increasing the frequency (speed) setting one increment. *Some people will be able to increase the amount of WBV much faster than other people. If you find that you are feeling better following the beginner's program, then you can increase your time and speed more rapidly.*

DAY 2: Increase the time by thirty to sixty seconds, staying at the same low speed. More sensitive people should do the same amount of time for two to five days before increasing, and then increase the time by only thirty seconds each session thereafter.

EACH FOLLOWING DAY (or every two to three days): Increase the time by thirty to sixty seconds, up to ten minutes, without increasing the speed.

- When you get to ten minutes, drop the time down to three to four minutes but increase the speed one setting.

Increase the time at this new speed following the same guidelines as above.

- As you gradually increase the speed, one setting at a time, follow this same pattern of increasing the amount of time day by day. Continue to drop the time back down when you increase the speed setting.

FAQs

Q. Can I use my vibration machine more than once a day?

A. Yes, but the total amount of time per day needs to stay the same. In other words, if you have been slowly building up and are now doing ten minutes per day without any problems, you can split that into a five-minute morning session and a five-minute evening session. You cannot suddenly start doing ten minutes morning and night without risking overdosing on your vibration.

Q. Does it matter what time of the day I use my machine?

A. Many people love to use the vibration in the morning to wake themselves up and set themselves up for a great day. Others might want to split up their time during the day for quick rejuvenating breaks. Some people find that an evening session is just the ticket for relaxing and helping them to sleep. Any of these approaches are fine. However, some people find that vibrating in the evening is too stimulating for them, and they have trouble falling asleep afterward—so if you try that and it doesn't work for you, no harm done; just do your vibration earlier in the day.

Q. Why does my nose (ear, feet, or any other body part) get itchy while I am vibrating?

A. We don't really know, but there are theories. One theory is that the increase in blood coming to the surface of the skin, due to an increase in circulation, causes itchiness. Another theory is that the itchiness could be a type of detoxing or energetic effect. The good news is that as long as the itching is temporary and goes away shortly after you stop vibrating, it is just a temporary annoyance and nothing to worry about.

Troubleshooting

- If you feel worse in the twenty-four hours after your vibration session, try less time and/or frequency the next time. You can even rest a day, and then only vibrate two to three times per week. Another good way to slow down is to just sit next to the machine and put only your feet on the vibrating plate.

- Don't forget to incorporate the other methods in this book for the best results lowering pain and inflammation! If you are having trouble, be sure to check out the chapters on gut flora and detoxing (chapters 8 and 9). It is common to overdo the vibration, leading to too much detoxification, putting undue stress on your liver, which temporarily weakens your immune system. As your liver is an important part of your immune system, this can result in a flare-up of gut flora issues. Gut flora issues can cause problems all over the body, so an increase in joint pain or headaches, as well as gut symptoms and many other issues, might be due to this phenomenon.

Advanced Program

Whole body vibration exercise is much more intense than conventional exercise. Workout times can be drastically shortened—with a very powerful machine, you can accomplish the same results in ten to fifteen minutes that would take you sixty minutes with conventional exercise. This is true because WBV requires your body to constantly respond to the rapidly moving platform beneath you, and the combined effects of gravitation, acceleration, and mass increase the amount of work being done. As my machines are gentler than the original Olympic-athlete machines, it is probably closer to a fifteen-to-sixty-minute ratio—but still an intense workout and an exciting thought! After you have acclimated to WBV and are feeling up to a more intense workout, you can maximize the muscle, bone, and other health and wellness benefits by following the training tips below.

You can work out daily with your vibration machine. WBV raises human growth hormone (HGH) and other hormones and brain chemicals that give you energy, which can help you recover from a workout and feel strong. If you are doing intensive daily training, you should vary the part of your body that you are focusing on.

Four factors determine how effective and challenging your training sessions will be:

1. the frequency (rate of vibration)

2. the position or posture you assume

3. the amount of time you spend holding a given position

4. the amount of weight you are supporting on the plate (if you want a more challenging workout, hold additional exercise weights)

Static versus Dynamic Exercises

It is important to note here that exercises can be done statically or dynamically. Static exercises are more appropriate for beginners or when starting to rehabilitate from an injury. Dynamic exercises are great if you are looking to make an exercise more challenging.

- Static exercise: Holding a pose in a position without moving while the WBV machine is on
- Dynamic exercise: Moving while the WBV machine is on (e.g., doing push-ups or squats)

Progressive Training Plan

I recommend progressively phasing in the following elements to increase the difficulty of your workout. As your body adapts and grows stronger, you can continue to challenge yourself with these methods.

1. Extend the time of each exercise.
2. Reduce the rest period between exercises.
3. Increase the number of sets per exercise.
4. Perform exercises statically (standing still), then dynamically (moving).
5. Add more challenging exercises.
6. Increase the frequency (Hz).

7. Incorporate unilateral exercises (perform exercises on one leg).
8. Incorporate holding increasing amounts of additional weight.

Ten Sample Exercise Positions, Massages, and Stretches

There are as many positions possible on the vibration plate as you can think of. Anything is fine; experiment and see what feels good. The following ten positions are a small selection of many possibilities. The first photo shows you a beginner's position on the Vibrant Health Gentle 500 machine. The succeeding photos are with the Vibrant Health Power 1000 machine, which is better suited for workouts and holding different positions. For more ideas, check out the poster available on my website, BCVibrantHealth.com, and that comes with Vibrant Health machines.

Exercise positions target different areas of the body, and some exercises target several areas of the body at the same time. There are leg, hip, and buttock exercises; arm, chest, and shoulder exercises; and abdominal and core exercises, as well as stretches and massages. Below are some of each of these different types of positions.

The muscle-strengthening effect is greatest when holding the exercise positions, but even if you just stand on the vibrating plate, you will still be getting many benefits. Even though exercises often target specific areas, many exercises will also be using other muscles all over your body to some degree. Some positions focus on one side of the body at a time; when you do these, to keep things even, you should also mirror image the position and do the other side, too.

For static exercises, you get into a position and hold it. For more intensive, dynamic exercises, you can move slowly in and out of the position.

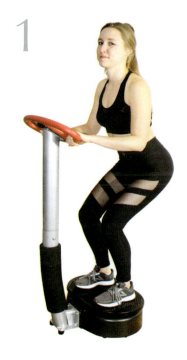

Beginner's position (Vibrant Health Gentle 500): Stand in a comfortable, balanced position with knees slightly flexed. If you enjoy the sensation of the vibration, you can straighten your legs, and more vibration will travel up through your bones to your entire body. If you don't like the vibration in your head, keep your knees bent. Hold onto a balance aid as needed.

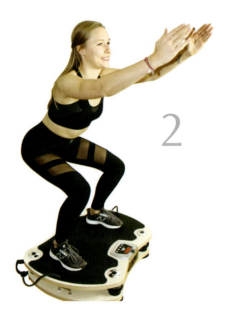

Deep squat (Vibrant Health Power 1000): Position your feet in the middle of the plate, slightly apart. Bend your knees about eighty degrees. Don't let your knees extend beyond your toes. Arch your back, keep your head up, and maintain balance. This position feels sort of like beginning to sit in a chair, then holding that position.

Pelvic bridge: Place feet on plate, slightly apart. Rest shoulders and head on the floor, extend your arms along your sides. Lift your hips and hold in your stomach.

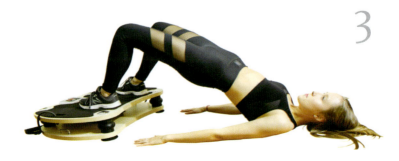

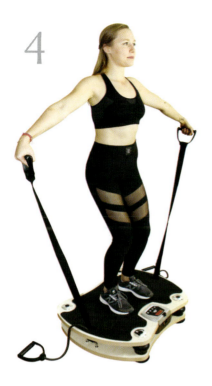

Lateral side raise: Stand upright on the platform and, with arms stretched out to the sides, pull up on the adjustable-length cloth straps.

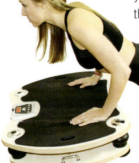

Beginner's push-up: Facing the plate, put your hands flat on the outer edges and keep your knees on the ground behind the plate. Line up your shoulders over your hands and pull in your stomach. Make a straight line from shoulders to knees. Bend your elbows to hold your weight. The more you bend your elbows, the harder this exercise will be.

6

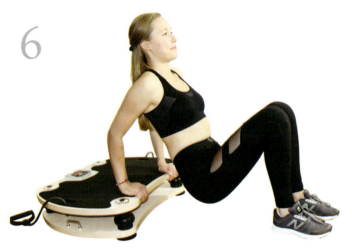

Triceps dip: With your back to the plate, place your hands at the front of the plate, shoulder width apart, pointing forward. Keeping your heels on the ground, bend your knees ninety degrees. Hold your waist in, keep your back straight and your head up. Lower your buttocks by bending your elbows and either hold that position or move up and down.

Diagonal crunch: Sit lengthwise on the platform. Bend one knee while straightening the other leg. Bring your hands to ears and bend your elbows. Touch your opposite elbow to the bent knee and hold while tensing your abdominal muscles.

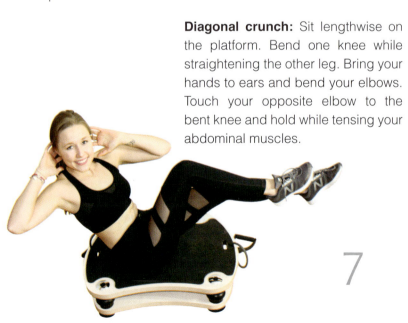

Hamstring stretch: Stand on the center of the plate with your feet together, knees slightly bent. Bend at the waist and grasp your ankles. This position stretches the hamstring muscles in the back of your upper legs.

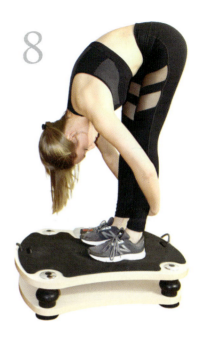

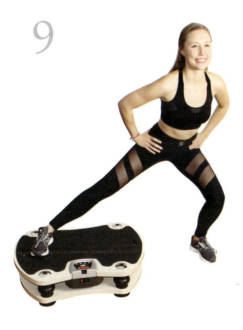

Adductor stretch: Stand beside the plate, facing forward. Place one foot on the plate, toward the back of the plate, so that your leg is stretched. With your weight on the leg on the floor, bend that knee and place your hands on your hips (or rest both hands on the bent knee). Slowly tense the inner thigh of the leg on the plate. This position stretches the muscles of your inner thigh.

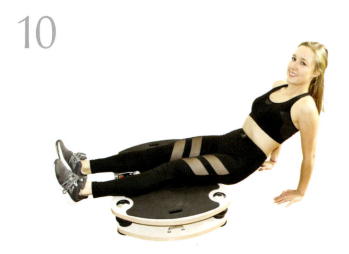

Hamstrings massage: Rest the backs of your thighs on the plate. Support your body weight on your hands. Hold your stomach in and keep your back straight.

Appendix 1

Vibrant Health Research Survey Summary

Effects of Whole Body Vibration Using the Vibrant Health Power 1000 in Retrospective Observational Survey[xix]

*Becky Chambers, BS, MEd.,
and Jaswant Chaddha, MD, FACOG
(unpublished data, 2019)*

Survey of People Who Use the Vibrant Health Power 1000 Machine

Specifications of the VH Power 1000 and method of use:

- Type of vibration machine: Relatively gentle, single motor, vertical vibration (entire plate moves in the same direction, up and down, at the same time)

[xix]Becky Chambers and Jaswant Chaddha, "Effects of Whole Body Vibration Using the Vibrant Health Power 1000 in Retrospective Observational Survey," 2019, https://bcvibranthealth.com/wp-content/uploads/2019/06/Vibrant-Health-WBV-Survey2019.pdf.

- Frequency = 26–45 Hz (increasing in 1 Hz increments)
- Becky Chambers's "Slow & Gentle" method

Metrics of Study Respondents

- 53 respondents out of 187 surveys sent out using HIPPA-protected online Survey Monkey website (28% response rate) in two weeks; no compensation was offered.
- 26% were 50–59 years of age, 62% were age 60–80, 2% were over 90 years of age. A total of 90% of respondents were over age 50.
- 58% female, 42% male
- 80% in average, good, or excellent health (self-rating)
- Most reported eating a healthy diet and taking few to no drugs.
- 55% of the respondents had had their machine one to two years, 43% for one to twelve months.
- Most had never used a vibration machine before.
- 64% reported following Becky's "Slow & Gentle" plan for starting WBV; 54% said this approach was important to them.

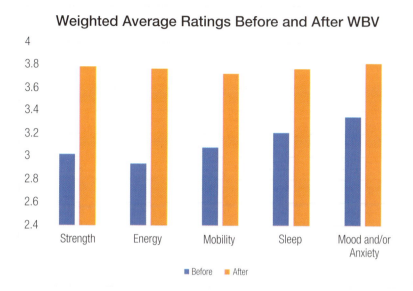

Five modalities—strength, energy, mobility, sleep, and mood/anxiety—were self-rated on a scale of 1 to 5, with "1" being weak/low/poor and "5" being very strong/high or excellent.

Improvements with WBV

Significant improvements were seen in:

Strength	25%
Energy	28%
Mobility	20%
Sleep	17%
Mood	14%

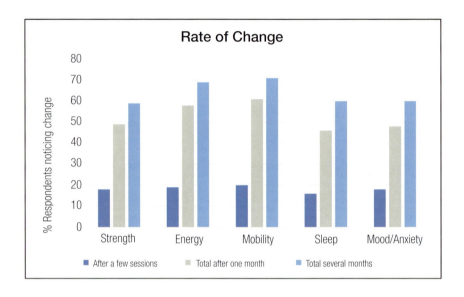

All modalities improved rapidly: strength, energy, mobility, sleep, and mood/anxiety.

- 15–20% improved after a few WBV sessions
- 45–60% total within a month
- 60–70% total within several months

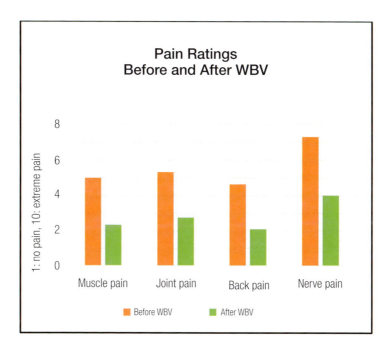

Thirty-nine respondents reported having muscle, joint, back, or nerve pain when they started vibrating. The average reported pain reduction, for all those reporting pain at the beginning of their WBV program, was 31 percent. Of those who reported an improvement in pain (74% of the 39 people who reported pain), their average reported drop in pain levels was 52 percent. Twenty percent of the thirty-nine respondents also reduced their pain medications after beginning WBV or switched to less powerful meds while reporting less pain. Most respondents took no pain medications.

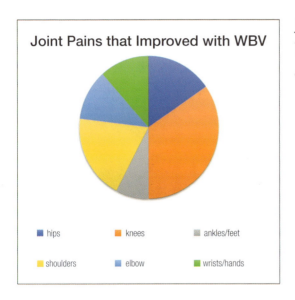

Joints all over the body improved, especially knee joints.

Pain relief was rapid for muscle, joint, back, and nerve pain. Most people whose pain improved noticed this improvement within weeks of beginning their WBV program.

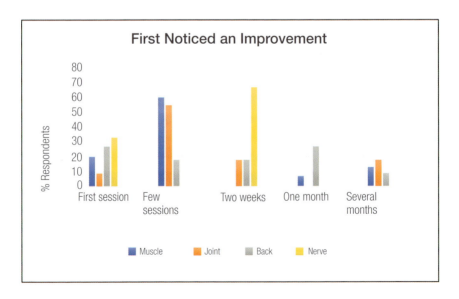

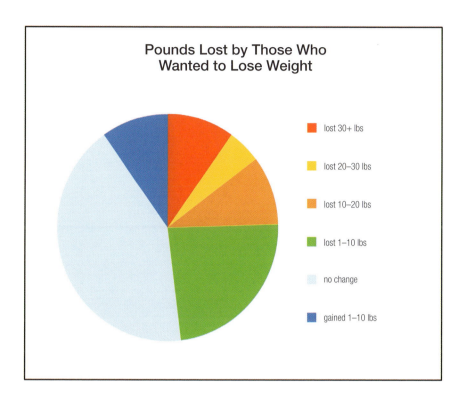

Almost half of those who wanted to lose weight did lose weight, ranging from a few pounds to over thirty pounds. Virtually all of the respondents (98 percent) were not taking weight-loss supplements or medications. Most followed healthy, low carb diet regimes, and 86 percent did not change their diets. There was very little change in the amount or type of other exercise for most respondents.

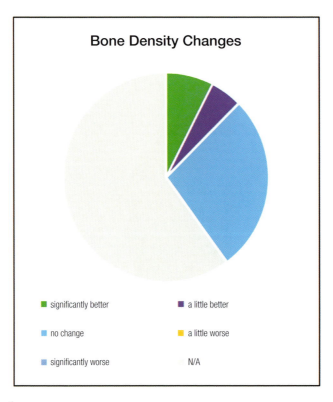

Bone density:
- 40% of respondents increased their bone density or did not lose bone density.
- 0% of respondents lost bone density.
- Considering that a large percentage of the respondents in this survey either already had osteopenia or osteoporosis, or were at high risk of developing low bone density, these results are excellent, indicating a reversal or interruption of the normal progression of this disease for 40% or more of the survey respondents.
- 60% answered Not Applicable (N/A): Most likely, many respondents had not used their machines long enough to have had a recent bone-density test and, therefore, were not able to answer to this question.

Vibrant Health Research Survey Summary

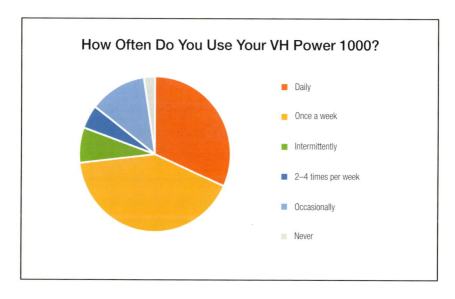

Seventy-three percent of respondents use their vibration machine at least two to four times per week. Only 8 percent use their machine occasionally or never.

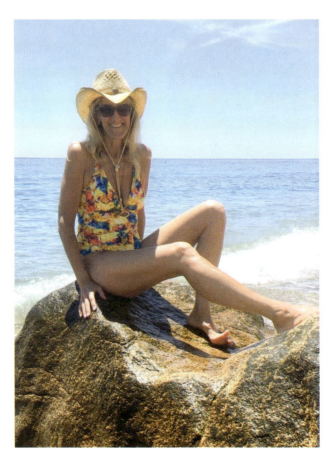

Becky Chambers, age 59

Appendix 2

Brain Synchronization

Brain synchronization is the simultaneous, in-phase firing of brain cells across regions of the brain. These combined signals generate electromagnetic brain waves, which can be measured by electroencephalography (EEG) and magnetic resonance imaging (MRI). Brain synchronization is associated with greater mental acuity and less stress. Since we know that lowering stress is important for lowering inflammation, it is not surprising that brain synchronization might also be associated with greater physical health.

How does this relate to WBV? Synchronized wavelengths from an outside source can cause "brain entrainment"—the synchronization of brain waves. This has been studied with sound and light and has been linked to increases in creativity, memory, learning, problem solving, and intuition, as well as to improvements in depression, anxiety, and ADHD.[xx] Biofeedback, for example, takes advantage of brain entrainment to treat mental

---

[xx] There have been many studies to back these claims. Please see the "Brain Synchronization" section under Additional Research Studies at the back of the book.

and physical health issues. There are now numerous companies promoting sound entrainment CDs for better brain function.

Synchronized brain waves seem to foster the formation of new synaptic connections, or brain plasticity, and learning. Earl Miller, the Picower Professor of Neuroscience at MIT and the senior author of a study published in *Neuron* in June 2014, has been studying the effects of brain synchronization. According to Dr. Miller in an interview with the MIT news office, he has found that "the phenomenon of brain-wave synchronization likely precedes the changes in synapses, or connections between neurons, believed to underlie learning and long-term memory formation."[1]

Brain plasticity (the formation of new connections between brain cells) has been known for some time to be a critical element for learning. However, brain plasticity, meaning the actual growth of neurons, takes too long to account for the human mind's flexibility. How the brain can process and utilize new information almost instantly has remained a mystery. As Miller explains, "Plasticity doesn't happen on that kind of time scale. The human mind can rapidly absorb and analyze new information as it flits from thought to thought. These quickly changing brain states may be encoded by synchronization of brain waves across different brain regions."[2]

Miller further describes the link between brain-wave resonance and brain development with an intriguing allusion to separate voices joining together; that is, waves of sounds: "There is some unknown mechanism that allows these resonance patterns to form, and these circuits start humming together. That humming may then foster subsequent long-term plasticity changes in the brain, so real anatomical circuits can form. But the first thing that happens is they start humming together."[3]

Brain synchronization also increases with meditation. Dr. Joe Dispenza, an internationally known lecturer, researcher, and author, has been studying and mapping the brain waves of meditators for decades. He describes the effects of brain synchronization, or coherence, thus: "What syncs in the brain begins to link in the brain. Once your brain gets coherent, you get coherent. When it gets orderly, you get orderly; when it works well, you work well."[4]

Dr. Dispenza describes the opposite state—that is, asynchronous brain-wave activity—as one that "causes our brain waves to fire in a very disordered, incoherent pattern (which in turn means our bodies can't work efficiently) . . . . the electrochemical messages or signals they are sending to different parts of the brain and body are mixed and erratic, so the body cannot then operate in a balanced, optimal state."[5]

Brain synchronization clearly has a great potential to affect our minds and lives, so I feel it is crucial to design and sell only vibration machines that produce a fully synchronized vibration for the best brain synchronization effect, as well as for a workout. I saw for myself the power of this effect early on in my WBV journey when I was using a double-motor vibration machine. Two motors cannot ever be fully synchronized, and thus will send a desynchronizing message into your nervous system and brain; over time, this was disastrous for me (see My Experience with a Double Motor Machine, page 143).

This is why all of the vibration machines sold through my company, Vibrant Health, are single motor only. A single motor produces a fully synchronized signal in the vibrational message going into your brain. I have now been using this type of machine for fifteen years with only positive effects; my body and mind are strong; in fact, my ability to create and communicate continues to grow as I reach out into the world with multiple books and a thriving company to share this revolutionary technology.

Appendix 3

FODMAP Diet Foods

Some foods are tolerated better than others. Therefore, the amounts of different foods are important, but there is also individual tolerance. This is an elimination diet in which you are first strict about eating only low FODMAP foods, then you gradually reintroduce foods to see which ones you can tolerate. People are still researching these foods and findings differ, so you should see also how you, personally, do with a food. Please also check with one or more of the FODMAP books in the resource section. There are also quite a few available on Amazon.

Low FODMAP Foods

- Protein: beef, chicken, eggs, fish, lamb, pork, prawns, and tofu
- Whole grains: brown rice, buckwheat, maize, millet, oats, and quinoa
- Fruit: cantaloupe, kiwi, limes, lemons, mandarins, oranges, papaya, rhubarb, and strawberries

- Vegetables: bean sprouts, bell peppers, carrots, choy sum, eggplant, kale, tomatoes, spinach, broccoli, Swiss chard, and all leafy greens
- Nuts: almonds, macadamia nuts, peanuts, pecans, pine nuts, and walnuts
- Seeds: linseed, pumpkin, sesame, and sunflower
- Dairy: cheddar cheese, lactose-free milk, and Parmesan cheese
- Oils: avocado oil, canola oil, coconut oil, olive oil, peanut oil, rice bran oil, sesame oil, sunflower oil, vegetable oil
- Beverages: black tea, white tea, green tea, peppermint tea, coffee, and water
- Condiments: basil, chili, ginger, mustard, pepper, salt, white rice vinegar, and wasabi powder

High FODMAP Foods

It is recommended that you avoid these. There are too many to list here, but comprehensive lists of these foods are available online (for example, http://www.myginutrition.com/downloads/High_FODMAP_foods.pdf) and in books.

Appendix 4

Severe *Candida* Yeast Overgrowth

I do not recommend starting out with a hard-core *Candida* yeast program. This could include avoiding *all sugars* (except for a few exceptions explained below). You would also need to be very careful about all products containing yeast, mushrooms, or mold. This results in there being a *lot* of foods you can't eat. This diet can produce dramatic improvements, but it is complicated, difficult, and restrictive. It can also result in a hyper-reactive state in which you can have major flare-ups of symptoms if/when you eat the wrong thing. This can create a serious situation and be quite scary if you already have health issues, especially if you are new to all this and don't have experience dealing with it.

If you have any potentially dangerous conditions, be sure to get guidance from a health care professional who is familiar with Candida *yeast before trying a hard-core* Candida *yeast program. You can also get guidance from the* Candida *yeast books listed in the resources section at the back of this book.*

In my experience, when properly using vibration—because WBV is so good for your immune system—many people will gradually heal from yeast with a simpler, more modified approach, as described in chapter 8. However, some people with severe *Candida* yeast overgrowths will feel better and benefit from a hard-core program.

If you want to try a hard-core *Candida* yeast diet, you should follow the guidelines in chapter 8, but you may also need to eliminate all fruit, not just high FODMAP fruits. You would also need to be strict about avoiding all foods that have yeast in them (such as bread, alcohol, vinegar, and fermented soy products), plus all foods containing these products. This is not easy to do, as these items are in *many* foods.

For example, vinegar is in many condiments, salad dressings, and mayo, which are, in turn, used in many other prepared foods. Yeast is used in seasonings (and not always identified; sometimes just lumped under the name "seasonings"), as well as in breads and other baked goods. Soy sauce is in many Asian foods. Molds are not only used to make some foods, like blue and brie cheeses and others, but also grows on leftovers in the fridge, so you would need to be careful about food storage.

Many people with severe yeast overgrowth may still be able to tolerate the safe sweeteners listed in chapter 8; however, some natural health doctors have told me that *Candida* yeast can adapt and learn to utilize these sugars as well, so they may not be safe for everyone.

Although some people may have trouble with any fruit when dealing with severe *Candida* conditions, they may be able to drink fruit juice consumed with the Special Diet Trick for Fruit Juice below. Dr. Keith DeOrio told me about this fruit juice trick many years ago when I had been dealing with extremely severe *Candida* yeast overgrowth for many years. I had not been able to eat any fruit for over ten years without becoming uncomfortably ill within hours. I tried this fruit juice trick and was amazed—no problems. I also saw my health improve immediately after adding fruit back into my diet, because fruit has many essential nutrients.

Particularly unique to fruit is its electrolyte balance. Electrolytes (potassium and sodium) in fruit are perfectly balanced for hydration (approximately 10:1), something no other food provides (most foods have more sodium than potassium and even vegetables have a ratio closer to 1:1). Our bodies are designed to operate with much more potassium than sodium. With our high salt diets and low fruit intake, many people end up with too much sodium and too little potassium, which can create major difficulties for hydration.

- *Diet Trick for Fruit Juice:* Fruit juice contains fructose, a type of sugar that will not raise insulin levels[1] or cause any other problems for most people, and it comes with a boost of essential nutrients in just the right balance for your body—especially those essential electrolytes. If you have *Candida* yeast overgrowth, you need to limit eating whole fruit, but you still need the nutrients in fruit. Consumed as whole fruit, the sugar will feed the yeast. But if you drink fruit juice on an empty stomach (at least one hour before food or two hours after food), the sugar in the juice will be absorbed in the small intestine, before the fluid gets to your large intestine where *Candida* yeast primarily lives—so there is no feast for yeast. But if the juice mixes with other foods, the sugar will bind to the solid fibers and be pulled into the large intestine, where the yeast will feed on the sugar. Remember, for this trick to work, it is critical that the juice be consumed on an empty stomach—at least one hour before food or two hours after food.

A hard-core *Candida* approach is very complicated, but it can provide great relief and help for more severe situations. More guidance can be found in the *Candida* yeast books listed in the Suggested Reading section (see page 216), and many natural-medicine doctors are familiar with *Candida* gut flora issues and can help you.

Appendix 5

Contraindications

It is always advisable to consult with your physician before starting any exercise program. Ongoing research in the field of whole body vibration (WBV) indicates that it can lower inflammation and that many people can benefit from this form of exercise. However, if you suffer from any of the following contraindications, it is imperative that you discuss WBV therapy with your physician before beginning any training program with WBV equipment.

Please do not use any WBV device without first getting approval from your doctor if you have any of the following relative contraindications.

Relative Contraindications—meaning that with special care and treatment, these conditions can sometimes not be a hindrance to, and may even benefit from, WBV.

- pregnancy
- epilepsy (very mild and not needing to be controlled with medications)

- minor migraines (mild, infrequent, and not needing to be controlled by medication)
- gallstones, kidney stones, bladder stones (WBV can help small stones move out of the body, but large ones may get stuck, potentially leading to severe problems.)
- articular rheumatism, arthrosis
- acute rheumatoid arthritis
- heart failure
- cardiac dysrhythmia
- cardiac disorders (post-myocardial infarction [heart attack])
- metal or synthetic implants (e.g., pacemaker, artificial cardiac valves, recent stents, or brain implants)
- chronic back pain (after fracture, disc disorders, or spondylosis, a.k.a. degenerative disk disease, a.k.a. arthritis)
- severe diabetes mellitus with peripheral vascular disease or neuropathy
- tumors (excluding metastases in the musculoskeletal system)
- spondylolisthesis (a misalignment front to back of the vertebrae) without gliding
- movement disorders: Parkinson's disease, MS, cerebral palsy, and others
- chondromalacia of the joints of the lower extremities, osteonecrosis
- arterial circulation disorders
- venous insufficiency with *ulcus cruris*

- Morbus Sudeck Stadium II (or complex regional pain syndrome [CRPS])
- lymphatic edema
- postoperative wounds

Absolute Contraindications—meaning do not use any WBV device at all if you have any of the following or if you have any concerns about your physical health! Note: conditions for which absolutely no vibration can be tolerated—such as broken bones, recent joint replacements and implants, and others—be aware that vibration will travel through wooden floors. In these cases, do not sit or stand next to a powerful vibrating plate. A cement floor should be safe, as very little vibration will transmit through cement.

- acute inflammations, infections, and/or fever
- large gallstones, kidney stones, bladder stones (large enough to potentially get stuck in narrow tubes on the way out of your body)
- acute arthropathy or arthrosis
- joint replacements: You must wait six months after a joint replacement before using WBV. After that time, WBV is okay; the vibration will then improve the bond of bone to metal or other synthetic material.
- bone fractures: For simple bone fractures, after six weeks it is okay to use WBV. For complex fractures or those involving implanted metal plates or screws, you must wait eight to twelve weeks before using WBV. Please consult with your doctor regarding your particular situation.

- acute migraine
- acute or severe epilepsy (i.e., needs to be controlled with medication)
- retinal detachment (or a high risk of retinal detachment)
- fresh (surgical) wounds
- implants of the spine
- acute or chronic deep vein thrombosis or other thrombotic afflictions
- acute disc-related problems, spondylolysis (stress fracture of the vertebrae), gliding spondylolisthesis, or fractures
- severe osteoporosis with BMD less than 70 mg/ml (T-scores less than −3.9)
- spasticity (after stroke, spinal cord lesion, etc.)
- Morbus Sudeck Stadium I (CRPS I)
- tumors with metastases in the musculoskeletal system
- vertigo or positional dizziness
- acute myocardial infarction

Notes

Chapter 1

1. Kris Gunnars, "Does All Disease Begin in Your Gut? The Surprising Truth," Healthline online, February 27, 2019, https://www.healthline.com/nutrition/does-all-disease-begin-in-the-gut.

2. Peter Boersma, Lindsey I. Black, and Brian W. Ward, "Prevalence of Multiple Chronic Conditions Among US Adults, 2018," *Preventing Chronic Disease* (September 17, 2020), http://dx.doi.org/10.5888/pcd17.200130.

3. M. Ariizumi and A. Okada, "Effect of Whole Body Vibration on the Rat Brain Content of Serotonin and Plasma Corticosterone," *European Journal of Applied Physiology and Occupational Physiology* 52, no. 1 (1983): 15–9, doi:10.1007/bf00429019.

4. M. Zago, P. Capodaglio, C. Ferrario, et al., "Whole-Body Vibration Training in Obese Subjects: A Systematic Review," *PLoS One* 13, no. 9 (September 2018): e0202866, doi:10.1371/journal.pone.0202866.

5. David Heber and Catherine L. Carpenter. "Addictive Genes and the Relationship to Obesity and Inflammation," *Molecular Neurobiology* 44, article 160 (April 2011), https://doi.org/10.1007/s12035-011-8180-6.

6. Teresa Carr, "Too Many Meds? America's Love Affair with Prescription Medication," *Consumer Reports* (August 03, 2017), https://www.consumerreports.org/prescription-drugs/too-many-meds-americas-love-affair-with-prescription-medication.

Chapter 2

1. Becky Chambers, *Whole Body Vibration: The Future of Good Health* (Charlottesville, VA: Quartet Books, 2013, 2020).

2. Ibid.

3. Becky Chambers and Jaswant Chaddha, "Effects of Whole Body Vibration Using the Vibrant Health Power 1000 in Retrospective Observational Survey," 2019, https://bcvibranthealth.com/wp-content/uploads/2019/06/Vibrant-Health-WBV-Survey2019.pdf.

4. M. Ariizumi and A. Okada, "Effect of Whole Body Vibration on the Rat Brain Content of Serotonin and Plasma Corticosterone," *European Journal of Applied Physiology and Occupational Physiology* 52, no. 1 (1983): 15–9, doi:10.1007/bf00429019.

5. Ibid.

6. C. Bosco, M. Iacovelli, O. Tsarpela, et al., "Hormonal Responses to Whole-Body Vibration in Men," *European Journal of Applied Physiology* 81, no. 6 (April 2000): 449–454, doi:10.1007/s004210050067.

7. Ibid.

8. Chambers, *Whole Body Vibration*, 56.

9. Elena Marín-Cascales, P. E. Alcaraz, D. J. Ramos-Campo, et al., "Whole-Body Training and Bone Health in Postmenopausal Women: A Systematic Review and Meta-Analysis," *Medicine* (Baltimore) 97, no. 34 (August 2018): e11918, doi:10.1097/MD.0000000000011918.

10. Bill Reddy, "Insights with Norm Shealy," *Acupuncture Today* 13, no. 6 (June 2012), https://www.acupuncturetoday.com/mpacms/at/article.

11. Ingrid Fadelli, "The Synchrony between Neurons in Different Brain Hemispheres Could Aid Behavioral Adaptation," Medical Xpress, June 18, 2020, https://medicalxpress.com/news/2020-06-synchrony-neurons-brain-hemispheres-aid.html.

Chapter 3

1. Mitch Leslie, "Good Vibrations: A Bit of Shaking Can Burn Fat, Combat Diabetes," *Science* (March 15, 2017), doi:10.1126/science.aal0919.

2. H. Yin, H. O. Berdel, D. Moore, et al., "Whole Body Vibration Therapy: A Novel Potential Treatment for Type 2 Diabetes Mellitus," *SpringerPlus* 4 (October 6, 2015): 578, doi:10.1186/s40064-015-1373-0.

3. Jack C Yu, Vanessa L Hale, Hesam Khodadadi, Babak Baban. "Whole Body Vibration-Induced Omental Macrophage Polarization and Fecal Microbiome Modification in a Murine Model," *International Journal of Molecular Science* 13, no. 20 (June 26, 2019): 3125, doi:10.3390/ijms20133125.

4. Direct email conversation with Dr. Yu, 2021.

5. Meghan McGee-Lawrence, K. H. Wenger, S. Misra, et al., "Whole-Body Vibration Mimics the Metabolic Effects of Exercise in Male Leptin Receptor-Deficient Mice," *Endocrinology* 158, no. 5 (2017):1160–1171, doi:10.1210/en.2016-1250.

6. Ning Song, Xia Liu, Qiang Feng, et al., "Whole Body Vibration Triggers a Change in the Mutual Shaping State of Intestinal Microbiota and Body's Immunity," *Frontiers in Bioengineering and Biotechnology* (November 2019), https://doi.org/10.3389/fbioe.2019.00377.

7. Dustin Heeney, Mélanie Gareau, and Maria Marco, "Intestinal Lactobacillus in Health and Disease, a Driver or Just along for the Ride?" *Current Opinion in Biotechnology* 49 (February 2018): 140–147, doi:10.1016/j.copbio.2017.08.004.

8. Ana Sandoiu, "Whole-Body Vibration Changes the Microbiome, Lowers Inflammation," *Medical News Today* (August 5, 2019), https://www.medicalnewstoday.com/articles/325948.

9. Ibid.

10. Yameena Jawed, Eleni Beli, Keith March, et al., "Whole-Body Vibration Training Increases Stem/Progenitor Cell Circulation Levels and May Attenuate Inflammation," *Military Medicine* 185, suppl. no. 1 (January–February 2020): 404–412, https://doi.org/10.1093/milmed/usz247.

11. Ibid.

12. Paula Rodriguez-Miguelez, Rodrigo Fernandez-Gonzalo, Pilar S. Collado, et al. "Whole-Body Vibration Improves the Anti-inflammatory Status in Elderly Subjects through Toll-Like Receptor 2 and 4 Signaling Pathways," *Mechanisms of Ageing and Development* 150 (September 2015): 12–19, https://doi.org/10.1016/j.mad.2015.08.002.

13. A. P. Simão, N. C. Avelar, R. Tossige-Gomes, et al., "Functional Performance and Inflammatory Cytokines After Squat Exercises and Whole-Body Vibration in Elderly Individuals with Knee Osteoarthritis," *Archives of Physical Medicine and Rehabilitation* 93, no. 10 (2012): 1692–1700, doi:10.1016/j.apmr.2012.04.017.

14. J. Bidonde, A. J. Busch, I. van der Spuy, et al., "Whole Body Vibration Exercise Training for Fibromyalgia," *Cochrane Database of Systematic Reviews* 9 (September 2017): CD011755, doi:10.1002/14651858.CD011755.pub2.

15. H. Zafar, A. Alghadir, S. Anwer, and E. Al-Eisa, "Therapeutic Effects of Whole-Body Vibration Training in Knee Osteoarthritis: A Systematic Review and Meta-Analysis," *Archives of Physical Medicine and Rehabilitation* 96, no. 8 (2015): 1525–1532, doi:10.1016/j.apmr.2015.03.010.

16. Gerhard Schuler, Volker Adams, and Yoichi Goto, "Role of Exercise in the Prevention of Cardiovascular Disease: Results, Mechanisms, and New Perspectives," *European Heart Journal* 34, no. 24 (June 2013): 1790–1799, doi:10.1093/eurheartj/eht111.

17. Anson M. Blanks, Paula Rodriguez-Miguelez, Jacob Looney, et al., "Whole Body Vibration Elicits Differential Immune and Metabolic Responses in Obese and Normal Weight Individuals," *Brain, Behavior, & Immunity - Health* 1 (January 2020): 100011, https://doi.org/10.1016/j.bbih.2019.100011.

Chapter 4

1. Jack C. Yu, Jaclyn M. Yu, Dhairya Shukla, et al., "Pain and Management of Pain: A Clinical Review for Craniofacial Surgeons," *Sage Journals* 2, no. 2 (May 2021), https://doi.org/10.1177%2F27325016211009271.

2. Amy Myers, *The Autoimmune Solution: Prevent and Reverse the Full Spectrum of Inflammatory Symptoms and Diseases* (New York: HarperCollins, 2015), 77.

3. Y. Zheng, X. Wang, B. Chen, et al., "Effect of 12-Week Whole-Body Vibration Exercise on Lumbopelvic Proprioception and Pain Control in Young Adults with Nonspecific Low Back Pain," *Medical Science Monitor* 25 (2019): 443–452, doi:10.12659/msm.912047; B. del Pozo-Cruz, M. A. Hernández Mocholí, J. C. Adsuar, et al., "Effects of Whole Body Vibration Therapy on Main Outcome Measures for Chronic Non-Specific Low Back Pain: A Single-Blind Randomized Controlled Trial," *Journal of Rehabilitation Medicine* 43, no. 8 (July 2011): 689–94, doi:10.2340/16501977-0830; T. S. Kaeding, A. Karch, R. Schwarz, et al., "Whole-Body Vibration Training as a Workplace-Based Sports Activity for Employees with Chronic Low-Back Pain," *Scandinavian Journal of Medicine and Science in Sports* 27, no. 12 (2017): 2027–39, doi:10.1111/sms.12852; J. Rittweger, K. Just, K. Kautzsch, et al., "Treatment of Chronic Lower Back Pain with Lumbar Extension and Whole-Body Vibration Exercise: A Randomized Controlled Trial," *Spine* 27, no. 17 (September 2002): 1829–34, doi:10.1097/00007632-200209010-00003.

4. A. Elfering, J. Zahno, J. Taeymans, et al., "Acute Effects of Stochastic Resonance Whole Body Vibration," *World Journal of Orthopedics* 4, no. 4 (October 18, 2013): 291–8, doi:10.5312/wjo.v4.i4.291.

5. Bidonde, et al., "Whole Body Vibration Exercise Training for Fibromyalgia."

6. H. R. Bokaeian, A. H. Bakhtiary, M. Mirmohammadkhani, and J. Moghimi, "The Effect of Adding Whole Body Vibration Training to Strengthening Training in the Treatment of Knee Osteoarthritis: A Randomized Clinical Trial," *Journal of Bodywork and Movement Therapies* 20, no. 2 (April 2016):

334–340, doi:10.1016/j.jbmt.2015.08.005; Y. G. Park, B. S. Kwon, J. W. Park, et al., "Therapeutic Effect of Whole Body Vibration on Chronic Knee Osteoarthritis," *Annals of Rehabilitation Medicine* 37, no. 4 (August 2013):505–15, doi:10.5535/arm.2013.37.4.505; A. P. Simão, N. C. Avelar, R. Tossige-Gomes, et al., "Functional Performance and Inflammatory Cytokines After Squat Exercises and Whole-Body Vibration in Elderly Individuals with Knee Osteoarthritis," *Archives of Physical Medicine and Rehabilitation* 93, no. 10 (2012): 1692–1700, doi:10.1016/j.apmr.2012.04.017.

7. Ibid.

8. T. Tsuji, J. Yoon, T. Aiba, A. Kanamori, et al., "Effects of Whole-Body Vibration Exercise on Muscular Strength and Power, Functional Mobility and Self-Reported Knee Function in Middle-Aged and Older Japanese Women with Knee Pain," *Knee* 21, no. 6 (December 2014): 1088–1095, doi:10.1016/j.knee.2014.07.015; T. Trans, J. Aaboe, M. Henriksen, R. Christensen, et al., "Effect of Whole Body Vibration Exercise on Muscle Strength and Proprioception in Females with Knee Osteoarthritis," *Knee* 16, no. 4 (August 2009): 256–61, doi:10.1016/j.knee.2008.11.014; N. C. Avelar, A. P. Simão, R. Tossige-Gomes, C. D. Neves, et al., "The Effect of Adding Whole-Body Vibration to Squat Training on the Functional Performance and Self-Report of Disease Status in Elderly Patients with Knee Osteoarthritis: A Randomized, Controlled Clinical Study," *Journal of Alternative and Complementary Medicine* 17, no. 12 (2011): 1149–1155, doi:10.1089/acm.2010.0782.

9. Zafar et al., "Therapeutic Effects of Whole-Body Vibration Training in Knee Osteoarthritis."

10. Ibid.

11. P. Wang, X. Yang, Y. Yang, L. Yang, et al., "Effects of Whole Body Vibration on Pain, Stiffness and Physical Functions in Patients with Knee Osteoarthritis: A Systematic Review and Meta-Analysis," *Clinical Rehabilitation* 29, no. 10 (2015): 939–51, doi:10.1177/0269215514564895.

12. L. Terhorst, M. J. Schneider, K. H. Kim, et al., "Complementary and Alternative Medicine in the Treatment of Pain in Fibromyalgia: A Systematic Review of Randomized Controlled Trials," *Journal of Manipulative and Psychological Therapeutics* 34, no. 7 (September 2011: 483–96), doi:10.1016/j.jmpt.2011.05.006; Richard Gerber, *Vibrational Medicine: The #1 Handbook of Subtle-Energy Therapies* (Rochester, VT: Bear & Co., 2001); N. M. Dhanani, T. J. Caruso, and A. J. Carinci, "Complementary and Alternative Medicine for Pain: An Evidence-Based Review," *Current Pain and Headache Reports* 15, no.1 (February 2011): 39–46, doi:10.1007/s11916-010-0158-y; J. M. Day and

A. J. Nitz, "The Effect of Muscle Energy Techniques on Disability and Pain Scores in Individuals with Low Back Pain," *Journal of Sport Rehabilitation* 21, no. 2 (May 2012): 194–8.

13. Bill Reddy, "Insights with Norm Shealy," *Acupuncture Today* 13, no. 6 (June 2012), https://www.acupuncturetoday.com/mpacms/at/article.php?id=32580.

14. Richard Gerber, MD, *Vibrational Medicine*, 3rd ed. (Rochester, NY: Bear and Co., 2001), 53–56.

15. American Association of Acupuncture and Bio-Energetic Medicine, "Basic Explanation of the Electrodermal Screening Test and the Concepts of Bio-Energetic Medicine," http://www.healthy.net/scr/article.aspx?Id=1085.

16. Norman Shealy, *Soul Medicine* (Santa Rosa, CA: Elite Books, 2006), 206.

17. Ibid., 212.

18. Ibid., 213.

19. Ibid., 212.

Chapter 5

1. M. Zago, P. Capodaglio, C. Ferrario, et al., "Whole-Body Vibration Training in Obese Subjects: A Systematic Review," *PLoS One* 13, no. 9 (September 2018): e0202866, doi:10.1371/journal.pone.0202866; M. Ariizumi and A. Okada, "Effect of Whole Body Vibration on the Rat Brain Content of Serotonin and Plasma Corticosterone," *European Journal of Applied Physiology and Occupational Physiology* 52, no. 1 (1983): 15–9, doi:10.1007/bf00429019.

2. S. Mohammad Alavinia, Maryam Omidvar, and B. Catherine Craven, "Does Whole Body Vibration Therapy Assist in Reducing Fat Mass or Treating Obesity in Healthy Overweight and Obese Adults? A Systematic Review and Meta-Analyses," *Disability and Rehabilitation* 43, no. 14 (July 2021): 1935–1947, https://doi.org/10.1080/09638288.2019.1688871.

3. Becky Chambers and Jaswant Chaddha, "Effects of Whole Body Vibration Using the Vibrant Health Power 1000 in Retrospective Observational Survey," 2019, https://bcvibranthealth.com/wp-content/uploads/2019/06/Vibrant-Health-WBV-Survey2019.pdf.

4. Ariizumi, "Effect of Whole Body Vibration on the Rat Brain Content of Serotonin and Plasma Corticosterone."

5. C. Bosco, M. Iacovelli, O. Tsarpela, et al., "Hormonal Responses to Whole-Body Vibration in Men," *European Journal of Applied Physiology* 81, no. 6 (April 2000): 449–454, doi:10.1007/s004210050067.

6. Chambers and Chaddha, "Effects of Whole Body Vibration Using the Vibrant Health Power 1000."

7. Gina Kolata, "Low Buzz May Give Mice Better Bones and Less Fat." *New York Times* 30 (October 30, 2007), https://www.nytimes.com/2007/10/30/health/research/30bone.html.

8. I. Janssen and R. Ross, "Effects of Sex on the Change in Visceral, Subcutaneous Adipose Tissue and Skeletal Muscle in Response to Weight Loss," *International Journal of Obesity and Related Metabolic Disorders* 23, no. 10 (1999): 1035–1046; F. Yang, J. Munoz, L. zhu Han, and F. Yang, "Effects of Vibration Training in Reducing Risk of Slip-Related Falls among Young Adults with Obesity," *Journal of Biomechanics* 57 (May 2017): 87–93, doi:10.1016/j.jbiomech.2017. 03.024; A. Figueroa, R. Kalfon, T. A. Madzima, and A. Wong, "Effects of Whole-Body Vibration Exercise Training on Aortic Wave Reflection and Muscle Strength in Postmenopausal Women with Prehypertension and Hypertension," *Journal of Human Hypertension* 28, no. 2 (February 2014): 118–122, doi:10.1038/jhh.2013.59; A. Wong, S. Alvarez-Alvarado, A. W. Kinsey, and A. Figueroa, "Whole-Body Vibration Exercise Therapy Improves Cardiac Autonomic Function and Blood Pressure in Obese Pre- and Stage 1 Hypertensive Postmenopausal Women," *Journal of Alternative and Complementary Medicine* 22, no. 12 (2016): 970–976, doi:10.1089/acm.2016.0124; A. Wong, S. Alvarez-Alvarado, S. J. Jaime, et al., "Combined Whole Body Vibration Training and L-Citrulline Supplementation Improves Pressure Wave Reflection in Obese Postmenopausal Women," *Applied Physiology, Nutrition, and Metabolism* 41, no. 3 (2016): 292–7, doi:10.1139/apnm-2015-0465; B. Wilms, J. Frick, B. Ernst, et al., "Whole Body Vibration Added to Endurance Training in Obese Women: A Pilot Study," *International Journal of Sports Medicine* 33, no. 9 (2012): 740–743, doi:10.1055/s-0032-1306284; G. Severino, M. Sanchez-Gonzalez, M. Walters-Edwards, et al., "Whole-Body Vibration Training Improves Heart Rate Variability and Body Fat Percentage in Obese Hispanic Postmenopausal Women," *Journal of Aging and Physical Activity* 25, no. 3 (July 2017): 395–401, doi:10.1123/japa.2016-0087; C. Milanese, F. Piscitelli, M. G. Zenti, et al., "Ten-Week Whole-Body Vibration Training Improves Body Composition and Muscle Strength in Obese Women," *International Journal of Medical Sciences* 10, no. 3 (2013): 307–311, doi:10.7150/ijms.5161; R. So, M. Eto, T. Tsujimoto, and K. Tanaka, "Acceleration Training for Improving Physical Fitness and Weight Loss in Obese Women," *Obesity Research and Clinical Practice* 8, no. 3 (May–June 2014): e201–e98, doi:10.1016/j.orcp.2013.03.002; S. Alvarez-Alvarado, S. J. Jaime, M. J. Ormsbee, et al., "Benefits of Whole-Body Vibration Training on Arterial Function and Muscle Strength in Young Overweight/Obese Women," *Hypertension Research* 40, no.

5 (2017): 487–492, doi:10.1038/hr.2016.178; A. Figueroa, R. Gil, A. Wong, et al., "Whole-Body Vibration Training Reduces Arterial Stiffness, Blood Pressure, and Sympathovagal Balance in Young Overweight/Obese Women," *Hypertension Research* 35, no. 6 (2012): 667–672, doi:10.1038/hr.2012.15; M. E. Zaki, "Effects of Whole Body Vibration and Resistance Training on Bone Mineral Density and Anthropometry in Obese Postmenopausal Women," *Journal of Osteoporosis* (2014): 702589, doi:10.1155/2014/702589; D. Vissers, A. Verrijken, I. Mertens, et al., "Effect of Long-Term Whole Body Vibration Training on Visceral Adipose Tissue: A Preliminary Report," *Obesity Facts* 3, no. 2 (2010): 93–100, doi:10.1159/000301785; A. Figueroa, S. Alvarez-Alvarado, M. J. Ormsbee, et al., "Impact of L-Citrulline Supplementation and Whole-Body Vibration Training on Arterial Stiffness and Leg Muscle Function in Obese Postmenopausal Women with High Blood Pressure," *Experimental Gerontology* 63 (March 2015): 35–40, doi:10.1016/j.exger.2015.01.046; A. Miyaki, S. Maeda, Y. Choi, et al., "The Addition of Whole-Body Vibration to a Lifestyle Modification on Arterial Stiffness in Overweight and Obese Women," *Artery Research* 6, no. 2 (June 2012): 85–91, doi:10.1016/j.artres.2012.01.006; J. Adsuar, B. Del Pozo-Cruz, J. Parraca, et al., "Vibratory Exercise Training Effects on Weight in Sedentary Women with Fibromyalgia," *International Journal of Medicine and Science in Physical Education and Sport* 13 (2013): 295–305; B. Sañudo, R. Alfonso-Rosa, B. Del Pozo-Cruz, et al., "Whole Body Vibration Training Improves Leg Blood Flow and Adiposity in Patients with Type 2 Diabetes Mellitus," *European Journal of Applied Physiology* 113, no. 9 (2013): 2245–2252, doi:10.1007/s00421-013-2654-3; A. Bellia, M. Sallì, M. Lombardo, et al., "Effects of Whole Body Vibration Plus Diet on Insulin-Resistance in Middle-Aged Obese Subjects," *International Journal of Sports Medicine* 35, no. 6 (2014): 511–516, doi:10.1055/s-0033-1354358.

9. Zago et al., "Whole-Body Vibration Training in Obese Subjects."

10. Milanese et al., "Ten-Week Whole-Body Vibration Training"; Zaki, "Effects of Whole Body Vibration and Resistance Training"; Vissers et al., "Effect of Long-Term Whole Body Vibration Training"; Miyaki et al., "The Addition of Whole-Body Vibration to a Lifestyle Modification"; Adsuar et al., "Vibratory Exercise Training Effects on Weight"; Sañudo et al., "Whole Body Vibration Training Improves Leg Blood Flow"; Bellia et al., "Effects of Whole Body Vibration Plus Diet."

11. Vissers et al., "Effect of Long-Term Whole Body Vibration Training."

12. Wilms et al., "Whole Body Vibration Added to Endurance Training"; Severino et al., "Whole-Body Vibration Training Improves Heart Rate"; Milanese et al., "Ten-Week Whole-Body Vibration Training"; So et

al., "Acceleration Training"; Figueroa et al., "Impact of L-Citrulline Supplementation"; Miyaki et al., "The Addition of Whole-Body Vibration to a Lifestyle Modification"; Sañudo et al., "Whole Body Vibration Training Improves Leg Blood Flow."

13. Miyaki et al., "The Addition of Whole-Body Vibration to a Lifestyle Modification."

14. Janssen and Ross, "Effects of Sex"; Wong et al., "Whole-Body Vibration Exercise Therapy"; Alvarez-Alvarado et al., "Benefits of Whole-Body Vibration Training"; Figueroa et al., "Whole-Body Vibration Training Reduces Arterial Stiffness"; Miyaki et al., "The Addition of Whole-Body Vibration to a Lifestyle Modification."

15. Miyaki et al., "The Addition of Whole-Body Vibration to a Lifestyle Modification."

16. Yang et al., "Effects of Vibration Training."

17. Miyaki et al., "The Addition of Whole-Body Vibration to a Lifestyle Modification."

18. Wilms et al., "Whole Body Vibration Added to Endurance Training."

19. McGee-Lawrence et al., "Whole-Body Vibration Mimics the Metabolic Effects."

20. H. Yin, H. O. Berdel, D. Moore, et al., "Whole Body Vibration Therapy: A Novel Potential Treatment for Type 2 Diabetes Mellitus," *SpringerPlus* 4 (October 6, 2015):578, doi:10.1186/s40064-015-1373-0.

21. Mitch Leslie, "Good Vibrations: A Bit of Shaking Can Burn Fat, Combat Diabetes," *Science* (March 15, 2017), doi:10.1126/science.aal0919.

22. Yu et al., "Whole Body Vibration-Induced Omental Macrophage Polarization."

23. Bellia et al., "Effects of Whole Body Vibration Plus Diet."

24. Chambers and Chaddha, "Effects of Whole Body Vibration Using the Vibrant Health Power 1000."

25. Ibid.

26. Barbara Bolen, "The Role Dysbiosis May Be Playing in Your Health," Verywell Health online (updated August 14, 2019), https://www.verywellhealth.com/what-is-intestinal-dysbiosis-1945045.

Chapter 6

1. Amy Myers, *The Autoimmune Solution: Prevent and Reverse the Full Spectrum of Inflammatory Symptoms and Diseases* (New York: HarperCollins, 2015), 20–25.

2. John B. Furness, Wolfgang A. A. Kunze, and Nadine Clerc, "The Intestine as a Sensory Organ: Neural, Endocrine, and Immune Responses," *American Journal of Physiology-Gastrointestinal and Liver Physiology* 277, no. 5 (November 1999): G922–G928, https://doi.org/10.1152/ajpgi.1999.277.5.G922.

3. "Gut Troubles: Pain, Gassiness, Bloating, and More," *News in Health* (February 2020), https://newsinhealth.nih.gov/2020/02/gut-troubles.

4. Myers, *The Autoimmune Solution*, 61.

5. Ibid., 76–77.

6. Jessica Stoller-Conrad, "Microbes Help Produce Serotonin in Gut," Caltech online (April 09, 2015), https://www.caltech.edu/about/news/microbes-help-produce-serotonin-gut-46495.

7. Myers, *The Autoimmune Solution*, 76–77.

8. Ibid., 37, 77–86.

9. Ibid.

10. Martie Whittekin, *Natural Alternatives to Nexium, Maalox, Tagamet, Prilosec and Other Acid Blockers: What to Use to Relieve Acid Reflux, Heartburn, and Gastric Ailments*, 2nd edition (Garden City Park, NY: Square One Publishers, 2009), 4–6.

11. Julie M. Deleemans, Faye Chleilat, Raylene A. Reimer, et al., "The Chemo-Gut Study: Investigating the Long-Term Effects of Chemotherapy on Gut Microbiota, Metabolic, Immune, Psychological and Cognitive Parameters in Young Adult Cancer Survivors; Study Protocol," *BMC Cancer* 19, article no. 1243 (December 2019), https://doi.org/10.1186/s12885-019-6473-8.

12. Myers, *The Autoimmune Solution*, 121.

Chapter 7

1. Kathleen DesMaisons, *Potatoes Not Prozac: Simple Solutions for Sugar Addiction* (New York: Simon & Schuster, 1998, 2019).

2. Artemis P. Simopoulos, "Omega-3 Fatty Acids in Inflammation and Autoimmune Diseases," *Journal of the American College of Nutrition* 21, no. 6 (December 2002): 495–505, doi:10.1080/07315724.2002.10719248.

3. Emmanuel Letavernier and Michel Daudon, "Vitamin D, Hypercalciuria and Kidney Stones," *Nutrients* 10, no. 3 (March 2018): 366. doi:10.3390/nu10030366.

4. "10 Signs You Need Methylation Support," BioCare, https://www.biocare.co.uk/news/10-signs-you-need-methylation-support.html.

5. Franziska Spritzler, "10 Evidence-Based Health Benefits of Magnesium," Healthline online, September 3, 2018, https://www.healthline.com/nutrition/10-proven-magnesium-benefits.

6. Whittekin, *Natural Alternatives to Nexium, Maalox, Tagamet, Prilosec and Other Acid Blockers*, 184.

Chapter 8

1. Amy Myers, *The Autoimmune Solution: Prevent and Reverse the Full Spectrum of Inflammatory Symptoms and Diseases* (New York: HarperCollins, 2015), 194–195.

2. Amy Myers, "How Do I Know If I Have Candida or SIBO?" updated July 30, 2021, https://www.amymyersmd.com/article/candida-vs-sibo.

3. Takashi Uebanso, Saki Kano, Ayumi Yoshimoto, et al., "Effects of Consuming Xylitol on Gut Microbiota and Lipid Metabolism in Mice," Nutrients 9, no. 7 (July 2017): 756, doi:10.3390/nu9070756.

4. H. S. Mäkeläinen, H. A. Mäkivuokko, S. J. Salminen, et al., "The Effects of Polydextrose and Xylitol on Microbial Community and Activity in a 4-Stage Colon Simulator," *Journal of Food Science* 72, no. 5 (June 2007): M153–9. doi:10.1111/j.1750-3841.2007.00350.x.

5. Kauko K. Mäkinen, "Gastrointestinal Disturbances Associated with the Consumption of Sugar Alcohols with Special Consideration of Xylitol: Scientific Review and Instructions for Dentists and Other Health-Care Professionals," *International Journal of Dentistry* (October 2016): 5967907, doi:10.1155/2016/5967907.

6. Myers, *The Autoimmune Solution*, 194–195.

7. Ann Boroch, *The Candida Cure* (New York: Harper Wave, 2018), 6–12.

Chapter 9

1. "Chemical Body Burden," test results done on Bill Moyers by Dr. Michael McCally, http://www.pbs.org/tradesecrets/problem/bodyburden.html.

2. Amy Myers, *The Autoimmune Solution: Prevent and Reverse the Full Spectrum of Inflammatory Symptoms and Diseases* (New York: HarperCollins, 2015), 20–25.

3. Maria Elena Ferrero, "Rationale for the Successful Management of EDTA Chelation Therapy in Human Burden by Toxic Metals," *BioMed Research International* (November 2016): 8274504, doi:10.1155/2016/8274504.

Chapter 10

1. Ana Sandoiu, "Just 20 Minutes of Exercise Enough to Reduce Inflammation, Study Finds," *Medical News Today* (January 16, 2017), https://www.medicalnewstoday.com/articles/315255.

2. Mayo Clinic Staff, "Rev up Your Workout with Interval Training," June 23, 2020, https://www.mayoclinic.org/healthy-lifestyle/fitness/in-depth/interval-training/art-20044588.

Chapter 11

1. James Nestor, *Breath: The New Science of a Lost Art* (New York: Riverhead Books, 2020).

2. Becky Chambers, *Homeopathy Plus Whole Body Vibration* (Charlottesville, VA: Quartet Books, 2016).

3. Jim Robbins, "Ecopsychology: How Immersion in Nature Benefits Your Health," *Yale Environment 360* (January 9, 2020), https://e360.yale.edu/features/ecopsychology-how-immersion-in-nature-benefits-your-health.

4. Ibid.

Chapter 12

1. Keith DeOrio, *Vibranetics: The Complete Whole Body Vibration Fitness Solution* (Santa Monica, CA: self-published, 2008).

Appendix 2

1. Anne Trafton, "Synchronized Brain Waves Enable Rapid Learning: MIT Study Finds Neurons That Hum Together Encode New Information," MIT News Office online (June 12, 2014), http://news.mit.edu/2014/synchronized-brain-waves-enable-rapid-learning-0612.

2. Ibid.

3. Ibid.

4. J. Dispenza, *Becoming Supernatural: How Common People are Doing the Uncommon* (Carlsbad, CA: Hay House, 2017), 67.

5. Ibid.

Appendix 4

1. Rebecca A. Evans, Michael Frese, Julio Romero, et al., "Chronic Fructose Substitution for Glucose or Sucrose in Food or Beverages Has Little Effect on Fasting Blood Glucose, Insulin, or Triglycerides: A Systematic Review and Meta-Analysis," *American Journal of Clinical Nutrition* 106, no. 2 (August 2017): 519–529, https://doi.org/10.3945/ajcn.116.145169.

Resources, Suggested Reading, and Additional Research Studies

Resources

Whole Body Vibration Therapy, Natural Health Methods

Becky Chambers, natural health practitioner, homeopath, BS, MEd
President and owner, Vibrant Health, Inc.
Ms. Chambers is available for consultations. To work with her, please contact her through her website: BCVibrantHealth.com

Naturopathic Organizations, Functional Medicine, Integrative, and Complementary Health Care

American Association of Naturopathic Physicians
    www.naturopathic.org

Also, to find health care professionals near you who will include nutritional and other natural methods in your treatment plan, you can Google the terms *functional medicine*, *integrative health care doctors*, or *complementary health care doctors*. There are no organizations for doctors who practice these methods, as these terms describe general approaches to practicing medicine not a specific type of doctor. But doctors who use natural methods will often advertise using these terms, even often including them in the names of their clinics, so a Google search of them will lead to many possibilities.

Homeopathic Organizations

American Institute of Homeopathy
   www.homeopathyusa.org
www.homeopathyhome.com
   A comprehensive and international guide to homeopathy that has links to many other resources and websites.

Suggested Reading

Vibration Therapy

Chambers, Becky. *Homeopathy Plus Whole Body Vibration: Combining Two Energy Medicines Ignites Healing*. Charlottesville, VA: Quartet Books, 2013.

———. *Whole Body Vibration: The Future of Good Health*. Charlottesville, VA: Quartet Books, 2013.

———. *Whole Body Vibration for Mental Health*. Lexington, MA: Transformations, 2020.

———. *Whole Body Vibration for Seniors*. Lexington, MA: Transformations, 2020.

Gut Health and Cookbooks

It is hard to split these books up into separate categories. The subjects are so interrelated that many of these books cover multiple areas. Check the titles for details.

CANDIDA YEAST

Boroch, Ann. *The Candida Cure: The 90-Day Program to Balance Your Gut, Beat Candida, and Restore Vibrant Health*. New York: HarperCollins, 2018.

Bruner, Sondi. *Candida Cookbook for Beginners: 85 Recipes to Alleviate Symptoms and Restore Gut Health*. Emeryville, CA: Rockridge Press, 2021.

Chaitow, Leon. *Candida Albicans: Could Yeast Be Your Problem?* Rochester, VT: Healing Arts Press, 1998.

Crook, William. *The Yeast Connection: A Medical Breakthrough.* Berkeley, CA: Crown Publishing Group, 1994.

Trowbridge, John Parks, and Morton Walker. *The Yeast Syndrome.* New York: Bantam Books, 1985.

Wunderlich, Ray Jr., and Dwight Kalita. *The Candida Yeast Syndrome.* New York: McGraw-Hill, 1998.

Gut Inflammation, SIBO, and Anti-inflammation Diets

Calimeris, Dorothy, and Lulu Cook. *The Complete Anti-Inflammatory Diet for Beginners: A No-Stress Meal Plan with Easy Recipes to Heal the Immune System.* Emeryville, CA: Rockridge Press, 2017.

Cole, Will. *The Inflammation Spectrum: Find Your Food Triggers and Reset Your System.* New York: Avery, 2019.

Hultin, Ginger. *Anti-Inflammatory Diet Meal Prep: 6 Weekly Plans and 80+ Recipes to Simplify Your Healing.* Emeryville, CA: Rockridge Press, 2020.

Hyman, Mark. *What the Heck Should I Eat.* New York: Little, Brown and Company, 2018.

Lapine, Phoebe. *SIBO Made Simple: 90 Healing Recipes and Practical Strategies to Rebalance Your Gut for Good.* New York: Hachette Books, 2021.

Myers, Amy. *The Autoimmune Solution: Prevent and Reverse the Full Spectrum of Inflammatory Symptoms and Diseases.* New York: HarperCollins, 2015.

Symon, Michael, and Douglas Trattner. *Fix It with Food: More Than 125 Recipes to Address Autoimmune Issues and Inflammation: A Cookbook.* New York: Clarkson Potter, 2019.

Whittekin, Martie. *Natural Alternatives to Nexium, Maalox, Tagamet, Prilosec & Other Acid Blockers: What to Use to Relieve Acid Reflux, Heartburn and Gastric Ailments.* 2nd ed. Garden City Park, NY: Square One Publishers, 2009.

Williams, Carolyn. *Meals That Heal: 100+ Everyday Anti-Inflammatory Recipes in 30 Minutes or Less.* New York: Tiller Press, 2019.

The Gut-Brain Connection

Mayer, Emeran. *The Mind-Gut Connection: How the Hidden Conversation within Our Bodies Impacts Our Mood, Our Choices, and Our Overall Health*. New York: Harper Wave, 2016.

Perlmutter, David. *Brain Maker: The Power of Gut Microbes to Heal and Protect Your Brain—for Life*. New York: Little, Brown and Company, 2015.

Homeopathy

Cummings, Stephen, and Dana Ullman. *Everybody's Guide to Homeopathic Medicines: Safe and Effective Medicines for You and Your Family*. 3rd rev. ed. Los Angeles: J. P. Tarcher, 1997.

Hershoff, Asa. *Homeopathic Remedies: A Quick and Easy Guide to Common Disorders and Their Homeopathic Treatments*. New York: Avery, 2000.

Lennihan, Burke. *Your Natural Medicine Cabinet: A Practical Guide to Drug-Free Remedies for Common Ailments*. Cambridge, MA: GreenHealing Press, 2012.

Reichenberg-Ullman, Judyth, and Robert Ullman. *Prozac Free: Homeopathic Medicines for Depression, Anxiety, and Other Mental and Emotional Problems*. Berkeley: North Atlantic Books, 1999.

Natural Stress Relief

Cronkleton, Emily. "10 Breathing Techniques for Stress Relief and More." Medically reviewed by Daniel Bubnis, MS, NASM-CPT, NASE Level II-CSS. Healthline online (April 9, 2019). https://www.healthline.com/health/breathing-exercise.

Decker, Benjamin W. *Practical Meditation for Beginners: 10 Days to a Happier, Calmer You*. Emeryville, CA: Althea Press, 2018.

Nestor, James. *Breath: The New Science of a Lost Art*. New York: Riverhead Books, 2020.

Reuben, Aaron. "The Incredible Link Between Nature and Your Emotions." Outside online (June 11, 2019). https://www.outsideonline.com/2397694/nature-mental-health.

Robbins, Jim. "Ecopsychology: How Immersion in Nature Benefits Your Health." Yale School of the Environment (January 9, 2020). https://e360.yale.edu/features/ecopsychology-how-immersion-in-nature-benefits-your-health.

Sockolov, Matthew. *Practicing Mindfulness: 75 Essential Meditations to Reduce Stress, Improve Mental Health, and Find Peace in the Everyday.* Emeryville, CA: Althea Press, 2018.

Sullivan, Laura. "Calm Within: Music for Relaxation of Body and Mind." Belmont, CA: Sentient Spirit Records. Audio CD.

Additional Research Studies

Brain Synchronization

Abraha, I., F. Trotta, J. M. Rimland, A. Cruz-Jentoft, et al. "Efficacy of Non-Pharmacological Interventions to Prevent and Treat Delirium in Older Patients: A Systematic Overview. The SENATOR project ONTOP Series." *PLoS ONE* 10, no. 6 (2015): e1023090. doi:10.1371/journal.pone.0123090.

Danilenko, K. V., and I. A. Ivanova. "Dawn Simulation vs. Bright Light in Seasonal Affective Disorder: Treatment Effects and Subjective Preference." *Journal of Affective Disorders* 180 (July 15, 2015): 87–9. doi:10.1016/j.jad.2015.03.055.

da Silva, V. F., A. P. Ribeiro, V. A. Dos Santos, A. E. Nardi, A. L. King, and M. R. Calomeni. "Stimulation by Light and Sound: Therapeutics Effects in Humans: Systematic Review." *Clinical Practice and Epidemiology in Mental Health* 11 (June 26, 2015): 150–54. doi:10.2174/1745017901511010150.

Petrovsky, D., P. Z. Cacchione, and M. George. "Review of the Effect of Music Interventions on Symptoms of Anxiety and Depression in Older Adults with Mild Dementia." *International Psychogeriatrics* 27, no. 10 (April 29, 2015): 1–10. doi:10.1017/S1041610215000393.

Raglio, A., C. Galandra, L. Sibilla, F. Esposito, et al. "Effects of Active Music Therapy on the Normal Brain: fMRI Based Evidence." *Brain Imaging and Behavior* 10, no. 1 (March 2016): 182–6. doi:10.1007/s11682-015-9380-x.

Schwartz, R. S., and J. Olds. "The Psychiatry of Light." *Harvard Review of Psychiatry* 23, no. 3 (May/June 2015): 188–94. doi:10.1097/HRP.0000000000000078.

Shealy, C. N. "The Reality of EEG and Neurochemical Responses to Photostimulation: Part I." In *Light Years Ahead: The Illustrated Guide to Full Spectrum and Colored Light in Mindbody Healing,* edited by Brian Breiling. Berkeley: Celestial Arts Press, 1996.

———. "The Reality of EEG and Neurochemical Responses to Photostimulation: Part II." In *Light Years Ahead: The Illustrated Guide to Full Spectrum and Colored Light in Mindbody Healing,* edited by Brian Breiling. Berkeley: Celestial Arts Press, 1996.

———, R. K. Cady, D. C. Veehoff, M. Burnetti-Atwell, et al. "Effects of Color Photostimulation upon Neurochemicals and Neurohormones." *Journal of Neurological and Orthopaedic Medicine and Surgery* 17, no. 1 (1996): 95–96.

———, T. L. Smith, P. Thomlinson, and W. A. Tiller. "A Double-Blind EEG Response Test for a Supposed Electromagnetic Field-Neutralizing Device. Part I: Via the Clinician Expertise Procedure." *Subtle Energies and Energy Medicine* 9, no. 3, 231–45.

Sun J., and W. Chen. "Music Therapy for Coma Patients: Preliminary Results." *European Review for Medical and Pharmacological Sciences* 19, no. 7 (April 2015): 1209–18.

About the Author

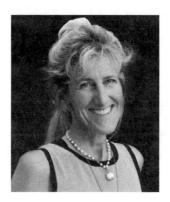

Becky Chambers is a natural health practitioner, teacher, author, and the president and owner of Vibrant Health, where she specializes in the breakthrough body, mind, and energy therapy of whole body vibration and the energy-medicine system of homeopathy. Chambers is a world expert in whole body vibration with twenty years of experience using and promoting it worldwide as an exercise and therapeutic system. Her bestselling book on the subject, *Whole Body Vibration: The Future of Good Health*, was released in 2013 and has been updated regularly. Chambers has a bachelor of science degree in biology from the University of Massachusetts, a master's in education from Lesley College, and she graduated from Clayton College of Natural Health in 2003 with a graduate degree in natural health, specializing in homeopathy.

She has spent the last thirty years discovering powerful new energy therapies, focusing particularly on whole body vibration and homeopathy, that have led to a transformation of her life on every level. She has published four other books: *Whole Body Vibration for Seniors*, *Whole Body Vibration for Mental Health*, *Homeopathy Plus Whole Body Vibration*, and a memoir (not currently in print), *Beyond the Great Abyss: A True Story of Transformation through Natural Health Breakthroughs*.

Becky Chambers is also available for consultations. To work with her, please contact her through her website at:

BCVibrantHealth.com.